Linda K. Fuller, PhD

Chocolate Fads, Folklore, & Fantasies: 1,000+ Chunks of Chocolate Information

Pre-publication
REVIEWS,
COMMENTARIES,
EVALUATIONS . . .

"**L**inda Fuller's new book, *Choco-late Fads, Folklore, & Fantasies* is WITHOUT A DOUBT THE MOST COMPLETE COLLECTION OF IN-FORMATION ABOUT THE CON-SUMING PASSION OF CHOC-OLATE. Not only is it complete, but it is delightful to read. I could have spent hours grazing its pages. It's a must for the devoted choco-phile."

Joyce K. Fuchs-Gioia,
formerly of Chocolatier;
President, J. K. Fuchs & Associates,
Marketing and Sales Consultants,
New York

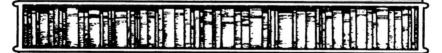

More pre-publication
REVIEWS, COMMENTARIES, EVALUATIONS . . .

"**J**ust as I was bracing myself to come out of the cupboard and admit my chocolate passion, I was relieved to learn that I am not a chocoholic, but a chocophile—that's much better! Thank you, Linda Fuller, for assembling this and hundreds of valuable tidbits for chocolate lovers long on the defensive. What is it about the psyche that we have to feel guilty about desiring wonderful things? Do we chocophiles lay guilt trips on you ascetics (who secretly love and maybe eat chocolate too)? No more bad mouthing chocolate! Read about chocolate's nutritive—even curative—properties and positive personality attributes of chocophiles. Enjoy dozens of wonderfully inventive chocolate confessions of famous and ordinary people. DR. FULLER HAS PUT HER RESEARCH SKILLS TO YUMMY ENDS, NOT ONLY IN GIVING US AN ARSENAL OF CHOCOLATE FACTS, BUT ALSO PROVIDING A CATALOG OF HOW TO GET AT CHOCOLATE IN ALL SORTS OF SOUL AND FANTASY GRATIFYING WAYS."

Marilyn Brownstein, BA
Senior Humanities Editor,
Greenwood Press,
Westport, CT

"**C**onsider this book a great gift box of chocolates, filled with morsels of delight meant to be savored over time. Roll the book around your tongue, let it melt into your psyche. Dip into it frequently, and it will surprise and delight you."

Martin Johner,
"The Chocolate Chef,"
Director of Special Events,
New School Culinary Arts Program;
Co-founder, Culinary Center
of New York

The Haworth Press, Inc.

Chocolate Fads, Folklore, & Fantasies

1,000+ Chunks
of Chocolate Information

Chocolate Fads, Folklore, & Fantasies
1,000+ Chunks
of Chocolate Information

Linda K. Fuller, PhD

The Haworth Press
New York • London • Norwood (Australia)

The Haworth Press, Inc., 10 Alice Street, Binghamton, NY 13904-1580

Library of Congress Cataloging-in-Publication Data

Fuller, Linda K.
    Chocolate fads, folklore, and fantasies : 1,000+ chunks of chocolate / Linda K. Fuller.
        p. cm.
    Includes bibliographical references and index.
    ISBN 1-56024-337-6 (acid free paper)
        1. Chocolate—Miscellanea. 2. Chocolate—History. 3. Chocolate industry. I. Title.
GT2920.C3F85   1993b
641.3′374—dc20   92-19440
                                                                                              CIP

This book is dedicated to my mother-in-law, who claims her love of chocolate began when her mother suggested she always carry it with her, "in case of an emergency."

Those of us who know Helen Smith Fuller claim we love her because she's always there and she's always real, she's a friend and she's a role model–whether for emergencies or for general chocolateering.

ABOUT THE AUTHOR

Linda K. Fuller, PhD, has written extensively about popular culture, including the tour book *Trips & Trivia*, an audience study on *The Cosby Show*, and a guide to *Community Television*, plus she is co-author of *Communicating Comfortably* and *Communicating Quotably*, and co-editor of the multi-volume series on American popular film, *Beyond the Stars* and *Communicating About Communicable Diseases*. Her other books for Haworth are *Yogurt, Yoghurt, Youghourt: An International Cookbook* and *Media-Mediated Relationships*. Dr. Fuller is an Assistant Professor in the Media Department of Worcester (MA) State College. She and her family, all devoted chocoholics, live in Massachusetts with their chocolate labrador retriever, "Truffles."

CONTENTS

Foreword

"From the *Chocolate Bible* to the Chocolate Hall of Fame"

In early 1982, while attending an antiquarian book fair in Greenwich Village, I had the occasion to visit Li-Lac's Chocolate Shop–to purchase chocolate, of course. In the front showcase, I noticed several copies of a book stored among an abundance of dark chocolate. The title of the book took me by surprise and I had to look at it, so I asked for a copy. The first thing I noticed was that the book smelled like rich chocolate. Little did I know at that time that this particular book would play an important role in my life, leading me into the world of contemporary chocolate lovers.

This richly scented book was *The Chocolate Bible* by Adrianne Marcus of San Francisco, with a dust jacket designed as a box of chocolates. It was full of all sorts of information, notably a list of chocolate shops from coast to coast. It was a real treat to read. Once I was home and my wife Emily read this *Bible* of chocolate we decided to contact Adrianne and obtain more copies to give as gifts. Through the course of corresponding with her and making plans to visit her in San Francisco that summer, I was introduced to friends of Adrianne's who put together festivals for food lovers and were planning a Chocolate Festival in New York City.

For this first Chocolate Festival in New York, as a guest of the Chocolate Manufacturers Association of America, I put together twenty displays of some of my chocolate graphics collection, representing the nineteenth and early twentieth century in Europe and America. I had been collecting historical prints, labels, posters, and advertising trade cards on or about the cocoa and chocolate industry for three or four years. Always a lover of chocolate, I clearly remember how good the chocolate Easter bunny was each year. When I became involved in the antiquarian book, print, and ephemera business, the natural course was to collect a particular favorite subject close to one's special interest. Since that time, I've become very involved with ephemera ("ephemera" are the minor documents of business history or social events which were printed or handwritten, to be normally thrown away once they were used), and I have been building a rather impressive collection of chocolate material. As a result, my collection has been drawn upon to be used for special articles and research, and I was honored to be one of the first inductees into the Chocolate Hall of Fame, back in 1990.

Chocolate Fads, Folklore, & Fantasies is a direct result of my visit to Li-Lac's and the purchase of my *Chocolate Bible*, when I introduced Eric and Linda Fuller to the topic.

Chocolate has been written about for over 360 years, but never has a culture been as influenced by it as ours has, beginning in the early 1980s, when chocolate in its many forms came to play such a significant role in our everyday lives.

William Frost Mobley
Chocolate Historian
Schoharie, New York

Acknowledgments

CHOCOLATE COMPANIES

Ambrosia Chocolate Company–Darlene C. Knuteson,
Sales Department
Au Chocolat–Pam Williams, Owner
Bakers–General Foods Consumer Center
Karl Bissinger's Chocolate Catalogue
Blommer Chocolate Company–Martin E. Krueger,
Vice President
Sydney Bogg Chocolates–Ralph D. Skidmore, Owner
E.J. Brach & Sons–Robert D. Hecklau, Senior Vice President
of Sales and Marketing
Peter Paul Cadbury, Inc.–Denis Dawson, Vice President
of Marketing
Chocolate Chocolate–Frances Park, Proprietor
Chocosuisse–D. Kuster, Director
Cocolat–Elliott Medrich, Owner
Cocoline Chocolate Co., Inc.–Joseph Kaufman, Director
of Marketing
Conadeca/Mexico–Jorge Fuentes Mercado, Director of Marketing
and Promotion
Cote d'Or–Christian Van Der Linden, Export Manager
Dilettante Chocolates–Dana Davenport, Director of Marketing
Double Truffle–Roman DeValenti, Owner
Fannie May–Susan V. Thorne, Assistant Vice President
of Marketing
Max Felchlin–Max Felchlin, Owner
Figi's, Inc.–Graham S. Alcock, Vice President of Marketing
Gabrielle's Fine Chocolates
Galerie au Chocolat–Stanley S. Thune, President
Ghiradelli Chocolate Co.–Dennis T. DeDomenico,
General Manager

Godiva Chocolatier–Holly Falken, Public Relations
Grand Finale–Barbara Holzrichter, Proprietor
Michel Guerard–Albert Pechenik, President
Guittard Chocolate Company
Harbor Sweets–Ben Strohecker, Owner
Hauser Chocolatier
L. S. Heath & Sons, Inc.–Sherry Foote, Public Relations Manager
Home of the Hebert Candies, Inc.–Frederick Hebert, Owner
Hershey Chocolate Company–Jay F. Carr, Vice President
    of Marketing
Holland Food Products–Tom F. M. Cuppen, Export Manager
Hooper's Candies–Barbara Bush Hooper, Owner
Hooten Chocolate Company–Gary Cestone, Sales Manager
Huwyler–Ward Ricke, Assistant Manager
Imports Unlimited–Nancy Carpenter Cook, Owner
Kosher Chocolate Factory–Philip Gelman, Owner
Kron Chocolatier–Tom Kron, Owner
Liled's Candy Kitchen–C. Henry Barner, Proprietor
Lindt & Sprungli, Ltd.–Dr. Rudolph K. Sprungli, Jr., Owner
Lisa Lerner Chocolates
Harry London's Candies, Inc.–Cedric Waggoner, Director
    of Marketing
Luden's, Inc.–Alfred Ciaramella, Director of Marketing
M&M/Mars–Elizabeth M. Kinney, Public Affairs Supervisor
Le Chocolatier Manon–Barbara Dubin, Vice President of Sales
    and Marketing
Madame Chocolate–Arthur "Jerry" Spiegel, Director
    of Marketing
Munson's Candy Kitchen–Bob Munson, Owner
Chocolatier Neuhaus–Yadja Zeltman, Director of Marketing
The Nestle Company, Inc.–Marie-Claude Stockl, Director
    of Public and Consumer Affairs (also, Eric Whiteway)
Perugina Chocolates–Matthew Glass, Public Relations
Poulain Chocolat Confiserie–Bethann Colle, Product Manager
Rebecca Ruth Candy, Inc.–John C. Booe, President
Red Tulip Chocolates Pty–Peter Salton, Director of Marketing
Regina's Fine Candies–Elliott Family, Owners

Rocky Mountain Chocolate Factory, Inc.–Thomas N. Hansen,
Director of Marketing
Ronsvalle's Candies–Gladys Ronsvalle
San Francisco Chocolate Company–Willis Good, Director
of Marketing
Miss Saylor's Candies–Jennifer Olmstead and Vicki Marinelli,
Directors of Marketing
Laura Secord/Confiserie Smiles Confectionery–Brian K.
Harrison, Marketing Manager
See's Candy Shops–Donald K. Hawley, Administrative
Coordinator of Advertising and Public Relations
Lee Sims Chocolates
Stork's Pastry Shop, Inc.–Karl Stork, President
Sucrs. de Pedro Cortes, Inc.–Norma Sanchez, Director
of Marketing
Tobler-Suchard, USA–Peter Baenninger, Marketing Manager
Sweet Swiss, European Specialties, Inc.
E. A. Tosi & Sons–Ernie Tosi, Jr., Director of Marketing
Van Leer Chocolate Corporation–Malcolm Campbell, Executive
Vice President
Vicki's Fine Chocolates–Vicki Fioranelli, Owner
Whitman's Chocolates–Demar R. Moeller, Director of Marketing
Wilbur Chocolate Company–James Maddox, Director
of Marketing
C & J Wilenborg, Inc.–Ernst H. Linnemann, National Sales
Manager
Willwood Group/Dublin–J. J. Fagan, General Manager for Sales
World's Finest Chocolate, Inc.–Frank J. Nudd, Vice President
Milton York Fine Candies

Chocolate-Related Companies and Persons

Boulder Calendar Company–Greg Amorese, Marketing
and Promotions
Ray Broekel–Chocolate Bar Historian
Candy Wholesaler–Shelley Grossman, Editor and Publisher
Chocolate Letter–Melvin Schechter, President
Chocolate Manufacturers Association of the U.S.A.–Richard T.
O'Connell, President

Chocolate News–Milton Zelman, Publisher
Chocolate Photos–Victor Syrmis, President
Chocolatier–Joyce K. Fuchs, Director of Promotion
Conadeca, the Mexican Chocolate Trade Organization
Culinary Center of New York–Gary Goldberg, Director
Dallas Alice, Inc.–Joan Rozansky, Director of Marketing
Dreams Come True–Aly Abrams, President
Dudley, Anderson, and Yutzy–Lenore Cooney
Ebullience–Myron Hankin, President and Owner
Holland Handicrafts–Adrienne Trouw, Owner
Journeyworld International Ltd.–Usha Menon
Marge Kehoe–International Cake Exploration Society (ICES)
Mohonk Mountain House–Carol Schimmer, Program Director
Mauna Kea Beach–Adi W. Kohler, General Manager
Pink Imports, Inc.–Sophie Dutordoir, Director of Marketing
Risk Enterprises–Brian Fenderbosch, Owner
Stouffer Westchester Hotel–Val Voelker, Director
    of Sales/Marketing
Swiss National Tourist Office
Uncommon Boston–Susan G. Berk, President
UAI Productions–Nancy Cummins and Karen Webber, Owners

Family and Friends

Alice Carter, for *Wall Street Journal* articles and Friday sherry
Marilyn Bugg Cooper, for accompanying me to Switzerland
Max Felchlin, for his generous philosophy on chocolate and life
Carol Frakes, for her freelance piece on chocolate psychology
Joyce K. Fuchs, for going way beyond *Chocolatier*
Fullers all, for being there and for loving chocolate
Suzanne Garber, for Western New England College library
    resources
Ginny Hersman, for Wilbraham Public Library resources
Gerard F. Keating, for monitoring the *Boston Globe*
Sarah Knutson, for the original Chocolate Orgy
Denise Marcil, for persisting that this get published
Genya Markon, for information on Israeli chocolate
Bill and Emily Mobley, for the festival, the feasts, the ephemera
Dr. Molly Noonan, for her medical dictionary

Jean O'Connell, for a great article on the Grand Chocolate Event
Bunny and Chuck Porter-Shirley, for Kentucky Colonels
Sue Russell, for catching the California chocolate scene
Rudy Sprungli, for lunch and laughs in Zurich
Henk Van Dam, for information on Dutch chocolate
  manufacturers
Everyone who salivated about and supported this project . . .

Chocolate is a perfect food, as wholesome as it is delicious, a beneficent restorer of exhausted power; but its quality must be good, and it must be carefully prepared. It is highly nourishing and easily digested, and is fitted to repair wasted strength, preserve health, and prolong life. It agrees with dry temperaments and convalescents; with mothers who nurse their children; with those whose occupations oblige them to undergo severe mental strains; with public speakers, and with all those who give to work a portion of the time needed for sleep. It soothes both stomach and brain, and for this reason, as well as for others, it is the best friend of those engaged in literary pursuits.

–Baron Justus von Liebig (1803–1873),
German chemist and dietetic expert

Chapter I

Introduction

This book deals with the "chocolate phenomenon" that is characterized by our going from buying 25-cent chocolate candy bars to spending more than $25 per pound for gourmet/designer chocolates.

THE CHOCOLATE PHENOMENON

Americans are on a chocolate binge. Last year alone, we spent nearly $6.7 billion on the industry.[1] Chocolate consumption in the United States is a healthy 2.6 billion pounds per year, up more than 20% since 1980. According to the Chocolate Manufacturers Association, per capita American consumption of chocolate is about 11 pounds per person.[2]

Chocolate is "in." It is everywhere, part of the good life. It is also part of Big Business. In many avant-garde restaurants, entrees are being pared and liquor sales are slipping, but gooey, irresistible chocolate desserts are being gobbled up at ridiculously inflated prices. Lush ads for chocolate are stuffed into upscale magazines, and nearly every major publisher has produced at least seven chocolate cookbooks in the last few years. At locations within walking distance and/or by mail order, we can fill our desires for chocolate delights ranging from imported Swiss ganache to freshly baked chocolate chip cookies, or even good old standbys like Snickers or Hershey bars. Throughout the country, chocolate-covered raisins remain the number one choice at movie concession stands.

Chocolate boutiques are sprouting up all over the place, featuring tempting choices like Dutch double chocolate truffles, Bavarian bonbons, chocolate-covered oreos, and various novelties ranging from the semi-practical to the outrageously kinky. You can go on a chocolate cruise, have chocolate tours arranged in major cities, belong to Chocolate-of-the-Month clubs, splash on chocolate scented perfume, indulge in chocolate binge weekends at participating hotels, attend chocolate festivals and fairs, decorate your clothes with chocolate sayings, enter chocolate sweepstakes, use chocolate in your fund-raising activities, and, of course, throw chocolate parties–or chocolate orgies, depending on your level of chocolateness!

There are also a number of services available that are chocolate-oriented. Some will execute your chocolate fantasy for you by appointment, while others can be contacted 24 hours a day to fulfill your chocolate needs. You can have your entire portrait reproduced in chocolate, or just your dentures ("The Ultimate Sweet Tooth"). You can have chocolate letters written for you, buildings sculpted for you in chocolate, or even have a chocolate FAX sent for you. If it can be done in chocolate, there is some enterprising firm out there doing it.

Chocolate novelties include just some of the following: chocolate pacifiers, chocolate tobacco, chocolate pill dispensers (maybe for your chocolate aspirin?), chocolate holograms,[3] or T-shirts with expressions like "Give me chocolate or give me death," "Open mouth, insert chocolate," or "Save the chocolate mousse." You can get a choco-bar biscuit for your dog, or chocolate lip gloss, chocolate pads, chocolate paper, chocolate bumper stickers, chocolate scratch-and-sniff labels. Do you like games? There's chocolate monopoly, chocolate chess, chocolate jigsaw puzzles, or chocolate dominoes; further, chocolate golf balls and chocolate tennis racquets are standard items. You can get chocolate packed in edible chocolate containers, or shaped like sexual organs. Choco-holics Unanimous puts out a "choco-holic" spray for those moments when you crave a quick chocolate smell. *New Scientist* recently reported on the Canadian Cold Buster,[4] a chocolate bar designed to combat hypothermia. Also available are: chocolate clothing, chocolate Christmas ornaments, chocolate pasta, chocolate soap, a men's cologne called "Hot Chocolate" (it comes packaged in a cocoa tin), chocolate coffee or chocolate tea, chocolate picture frames, chocolate subway tokens, chocolate use-your-imagination . . .

Not only is chocolate in the media (it has been noted that when a magazine has chocolate on the cover, sales double), 1983 saw the introduction of a publication for the gourmet chocolate lover: *Chocolatier* already has nearly one-quarter of a million subscribers. "Chocolate News," a newsletter declaring itself "chocolate central in the chocolate universe," chose chocolate-covered pages for its chocolate information.

Sandra Boynton's highly successful illustrated book, *Chocolate: The Consuming Passion,* sold 140,000 copies in the United States, and has been greeted around the world with equal enthusiasm. The cartoonist has also done quite a business with chocolate novelties like mugs, calendars, greeting cards, and her famous T-shirt that reads, "EMERGENCY ALERT. If wearer of this shirt is found vacant, listless, or depressed, ADMINISTER CHOCOLATE IMMEDIATELY."

In addition, Americans spend more than $400 million annually on fresh-baked, soft-and-chewy, over-the-counter chocolate cookies.[5] "Designer ice cream," mostly featuring chocolate, is also a multimillion-dollar industry. A craze for chocolate soda was set off with the success of Canfield's diet fudge soda, and its effects have hit the highly competitive and highly profitable global soft drink market. And still, consider this: some 20 to 25 million Hershey Kisses are produced each day.

It has been theorized that this chocolate phenomenon represents the ultimate Yuppie self-reward for these times. Yet chocolate, you will learn here, has long been our favorite flavor. The difference is that chocophiles and chocoholics have come out of the closet, encouraged and enhanced by any number of chocomarketing schemes.

IN THE BEGINNING . . .

The history of chocolate weaves stories of aphrodisiacs and apostles, inventions and intrigues, folklore and fantasies. It all began at least 4,000 years ago, when Egyptians displayed their confectionery pleasures on papyrus. There is documentation that sweetmeats were being sold in the marketplace as early as 1566 B.C. Yet chocolate itself didn't appear on the scene until the value of the cacao plant was discovered by ancient Aztec and Mayan cultures. Chocolate in the form of cocoa beans is reputed to have originated in the Amazon or Orinoco basin. The Aztecs and Mayans reportedly used the beans to make a potent drink they called "xocoatl."

Although they had been familiar with cocoa for several centuries, it wasn't until around 600 A.D. that the Mayans migrated into the northern regions of South America and established the earliest known cocoa plantations in the Yucatan. Cocoa had long been considered a valuable commodity, and the early Indian cultures used it both as a means of payment and as units of calculation. One hundred beans, it was said, could obtain "a tolerably good slave."[6]

Ancient chronicles report on the belief of the Aztecs that their principal god, Quetzalcoatl-Tlahuizcalpanticutli, who was symbolized by a feathered serpent, travelled to earth on a beam of the Morning Star with "cauhcacahuatl" (the cacao tree) from Paradise. In doing so, the god of light was thought to take his offering to the people. His religious doctrine was to inspire creative enterprise on the part of his disciples, and they were encouraged to begin harvesting the cacao tree.

It was from Quetzalcoatl the god-man that the Aztecs learned how to use cacao beans–how to roast and grind them, making a nourishing paste that could be dissolved in water. Quetzalcoatl, it was said, "was bearded and white-skinned, and he came from the Land of Gold where the sun rests at night. In the time before memory he was born of a god and a virgin mortal, endowed with all knowledge and wisdom. He had come down to Mexico to be the people's priest-king and to teach them the arts: painting and the working of silver, wood, and feathers. He had given the Aztecs their calendar, shown them how to grow maize. And from heaven he had brought the seeds of the cocoa tree. He showed his people how to grow the tree and how to make chocolate from it."[7]

The ancients then added spices to the cacao paste and called their special drink "chocolatl," meaning bitter-water. They believed that the imbibing of "chocolatl" brought universal wisdom and knowledge, which continued in the afterlife.

The ancient Mexicans also took it as a matter of faith that the goddess of food, Tonacatecutli, and the goddess of water, Calchiuhtlucue, were the guardian goddesses of cocoa. Human sacrifices were performed each year for these goddesses, with victims appropriately given cacao at their last meals.

In addition to using cacao as a food item, Mexicans also used its seeds as a medium of exchange. It is a part of the early record that, "In certain provinces called Guatimala and Soconusco there is growing a great store of cacao, which is a berry like unto an almond. It is the best merchandise in all the Indies. The Indians make drink of it, and in like manner meat to eat. It goeth currently for money in any market, or fair, and may buy flesh, fish, bread or cheese, or other things."[8]

"THEOBROMA CACAO"[9]

The actual term "chocolate" is said to have derived from a combination of the Mayan word "xocoatl," and the Aztec word for cocoa, "cacahuatl," meaning "food of the gods." The following "Ode to Chocolate," originally written in Latin in 1664 by a Jesuit priest, Aloysius Ferronius, was dedicated to Cardinal Francis Maria Brancaccio of the Vatican:

O tree, born in far off lands,
Price of Mexico's shores,
Rich with a heavenly nectar
That will conquer all who taste it.

To them let every tree pay homage,
And every flower bow its head in praise.
The wreath of the laurel crowns you; the oak, the alder,
And the precious cedar proclaim your triumph.

Some say you lived in Eden with Adam
And that he carried you with him when he fled.
And from thence you journeyed to the Indes
Where you prospered in the hospitable soil,
And your trunk burgeoned with
The bounty of your noble seeds.

Are you another gift of Bacchus,
Famed for his free-flowing wines?

No–the fruits of Crete and Massica
Bring not the glory you do to your native land.

For you are a fresh shower that bedews the heart,
The fountain of a poet's gentle spirit.
O sweet liquor sent from the stars,
Surely you must be the drink of the gods![10]

"Chocolate" is a Mexican-Indian collaboration of the terms *Choco* ("foam") and *atl* ("water"). The cocoa bean comes from the cacao tree, and our word for its ultimate food is "chocolate." Thomas Gage wrote in his 1648 "New Survey of the West Indies": "The name chocolatte is an Indian name, and is compounded from 'atta' . . . which in the Mexican language signifieth water, and from the sound which the water (wherein is put the chocolatte) makes, as 'choco, choco, choco,' when it is stirred in a cup by an instrument called a 'molinet,' until it bubble and rise into a froath."

The Swedish naturalist Carolus Linneaus (1707-1778) wasn't satisfied with the term "cocoa," and decided in 1753 to rename it "Theobroma Cacao," the Greek word for "food of the gods."[11]

In its early days, chocolate was solely consumed as a beverage. It was a standard part of the ritual in 12th century Mesoamerican marriages to share a mug of frothy chocolate.

Writing in 1923 about "The Cocoa and Chocolate Industry," Arthur W. Knapp discusses how, according to Mexican mythology, "Chocolate was consumed by the Gods in Paradise, and the seed of cocoa was conveyed to man as a special blessing by the God of the Air."

CHOCOLATE IS INTRODUCED TO THE WORLD

Credit for introducing chocolate to Europe goes to Christopher Columbus, who brought cacao beans back with him to King Ferdinand V and Queen Isabella of Spain from his fourth visit, in 1502, to the New World. Somehow, however, the importance of the little brown, almond-shaped beans was overlooked in favor of the many other treasures Columbus brought with him on his return. It has been recorded that, "At the discovery of America, the natives of the narrower portion of the continent bordering on the Caribbean Sea were found of two luxuries which have been everywhere recognized as worthy of extensive cultivation; namely, tobacco and chocolate."[12]

The big date on which chocolate was first noted was 1519, when the Spanish soldier/explorer Hernando Cortez visited the court of Montezuma, the Aztec emperor of Mexico. According to an account in American historian William Hickling Prescott's 1838 *History of the Conquest of Mexico*, Montezuma "took no other beverage than CHOCOLATL, a potation of chocolate, flavored with vanilla and other spices, and so prepared as to be reduced to a froth of the consistency of honey, which gradually dissolved in the mouth and was taken cold." No fewer than 50 jars of the beverage were prepared each day for Emperor Montezuma. As the story spread that Montezuma always drank his "chocolatl" in golden goblets before entering his harem, the notion was born that this special "chocolatl" was an aphrodisiac.

Cortez made careful note of the Aztec's methods of cultivating cacao beans, observing how the Indians roasted and ground them, then flavored the beans with various herbs and spices. By 1528 he and his Conquistadores introduced the Mexican chocolate to the royal court of King Charles V. The official report was this: "Un taza de ester preciosa brehaje peremete un hombre de andar an dia entero sin tomar alimento," which freely translated means that a cup of chocolate each day provided great energy. Spain was so enthralled with the powers of chocolate that it commissioned its special prize to some monks who, hidden away in Spanish monasteries, secretly processed the cocoa beans. The chocolate secret, amazingly, was kept for nearly a century! The Nestle Company's *History of Chocolate and Cocoa* discusses how in 1631 a Spaniard named Colmenero published a book called *A Curious Treatise Of the Nature And Quality Of Chocolate*, later translated into many languages and considered the standard work on the subject for about a hundred years. Besides being a delightful beverage, chocolate was also the source of a profitable industry for Spain, which planted numerous cocoa trees in its overseas colonies.

It was an Italian traveler—Antonio Carletti—who in 1606 discovered the chocolate treasure and determined to take it back to his country and beyond. The leak of the secret of cocoa coincided with the decline of Spain as a major world power, and the Spanish Crown's monopoly of the chocolate trade was finished. In just a few years, knowledge of its powers had spread through France, Italy, Germany, and England. The Duke of Alva[13] is credited with bringing chocolate from Spain to the low countries.

Brillat-Savarin's *Physiologie du Gout* (1825) recounts that in 1615, when the Spanish Princess Maria Theresa was betrothed to Louis XIV of France, she gave her fiancé an engagement gift of chocolate, which came packaged in an elegantly ornate chest. The marriage of Maria Theresa and Louis XIV serves as a symbol of the marriage of chocolate into the Spanish-Franco culture.

The sixteenth century Spanish historian Hernando de Oviedo y Valdez has written: "None but the rich and noble could afford to drink chocolatl, as it was literally drinking money. Cocoa passed as currency among all nations; thus a rabbit in Nicaragua sold for 10 cocoa nibs, and 100 of these seeds could buy a tolerably good slave."[14]

Besides being classist, the drinking of chocolate was also sexist, being a beverage predominantly served to men. The 1664 diary of Samuel Pepys records that "jocalette" was a very well-received item of the day.

On June 16, 1657, what is believed to be the earliest notice of the sale of chocolate in England, the following item appeared in the *Public Advertiser*: "In Bishopsgate Street, in Queen's Head Alley, at a Frenchman's house, is an excellent West India drink, called chocolate, to be sold, where you may have it ready at any time; and also unmade, at reasonable rates."[15]

CHOCOLATE HOUSES

By the middle of the seventeenth century, chocolate houses began appearing, the first one in London in 1657, opened by a Frenchman. Occasionally spices and flavorings like vanilla, cloves, cinnamon, or aniseed were added to give a fillip to the beverage. Soon, other cafes serving chocolate drinks sprang up in the Netherlands, France, Belgium, Germany, and Switzerland; later in the century, cocoa came to Austria and Italy.

Chocolate was considered *the* drink at the fashionable court of Louis XIV of France, and it took on its own sense of status as silversmiths and porcelain manufacturers were commissioned to create elegant chocolate services. Investment in cacao cultivation in the British West Indies began in earnest.

The story is told that Spanish ladies were so fond of chocolate that they sometimes had it brought to them at church, an act which was often reproved by the bishops.

At a cost at that time of 10 to 15 shillings per pound, chocolate remained a beverage for the elite class. By 1730, the price had dropped from the equivalent of about $3 per pound to at last being within the financial reach of persons other than just the very wealthy.

Writing about the introduction of cocoa, coffee, and tea into Europe, Isaac Disraeli[16] wrote the following in his six-volume *Curiosities of Literature*: "Chocolate the Spaniards brought from Mexico, where it was denominated CHOCOLATL. It was a coarse mixture of ground cacao and Indian corn with roucou; but the Spaniards, liking its nourishment, improved it into a richer compound with sugar, vanilla and other aromatics. We had Chocolate houses in London long after coffee houses; they seemed to have associated something more elegant and refined in their new form when the other had become common."

EATING CHOCOLATE

Chocolate in its earliest days, then, was best in liquid form–a process that wasn't easy to attempt at home. The Nestle Company has shared ingredients for a typical recipe[17]:

700 cocoa beans
1-1/2 lbs. sugar
2 oz. cinnamon
14 peppercorns from Mexico
1/2 oz. cloves
3 vanilla beans, or, instead, 2 ounces of aniseed
the biggest part of a hazelnut

By 1674, eating chocolate in solid form was introduced in Spain in the form of rolls and cakes, typically served in the various chocolate emporiums of the day. Soon, the habit took hold in London's "At the Coffee Mill and Tobacco Roll," and eventually chocolate "in the Spanish style" spread further throughout Europe.

Yet, it was to be another 200 years before Fry & Sons of England sold a product called "Chocolate Delicieux a Manger" in 1847, thought to be the first chocolate bar for eating (though not the first time chocolate had been eaten; it had been reported that "The virulently narcotic cocoa leaf is chewed by natives of the West Coast of South America").[18]

In 1849, an exhibition in Bingley Hall at Birmingham, England, Cadbury Brothers had a display of eating chocolate.

CHOCOLATE IN MEDICINE AND LAW

In addition, chocolate appears to have been used as a medicinal remedy by leading physicians of the day for any number of ailments. Christopher Judwig Hoffmann's treatise *Potus Chocolate* recommends chocolate for many diseases, and cites it in particular as a cure for Cardinal Richelieu's ills. As word of its powers spread, physicians began prescribing chocolate as a cure-all for their patients.

Chocolate is not only pleasant of taste, but it is also a veritable balm of the mouth, for the maintaining of all glands and humours in a good state of health. Thus it is, that all who drink it, possess a sweet breath," wrote Doctor Stephani Blancardi of Amsterdam in 1705.[19] Chocosuisse, the Union of Swiss Chocolate Manufacturers, shares this information: "During the 17th and 18th centuries, when whole books were written in praise of chocolate, there was hardly an illness for which chocolate was not prescribed as a cure, scarcely a sensory function whose improvement was not attributed to chocolate, and not a few of the leading figures of the time freely admitted that they owed a great deal to chocolate."[20]

The positive medicinal aspects of chocolate continued as a theme into the twentieth century. In an address delivered before the Cleveland Retail Grocer's Association in 1903, B. P. Forbes of the Forbes Chocolate Company gave this testimonial: "I have personal knowledge of two or three typhoid fever patients in hospitals in Cleveland, within the past few weeks, who have been allowed the use of Dutch cocoa from four to six times a day, and have recuperated rapidly on this diet. Cocoa nourishes and builds up the brain and muscle and may be safely used by any member of the family."[21] More recently, Dr. Joseph H. Fries has declared, "Allergists, dermatologists, gastroenterologists, dentists each have put forth reasons for the avoidance of chocolate in the diet. It is timely to try to separate truth from myth. To do so becomes important because chocolate is a highly nutritious food whose virtues have been recognized where high energy in small bulk is critical."[22] (Do you need any more rationalizations to enjoy chocolate? Wait until you get to the "Chocolate Nutrition" section of this book!)

Chocolate even made the law books: it is on record that in 1747 Frederic the Great of Prussia issued an edict forbidding the "hawking of chocolate."

DEVELOPMENTS IN THE NINETEENTH CENTURY

In 1795, Dr. Joseph Fry of Bristol, England, invented a steam engine that could grind cocoa beans faster, which meant that chocolate no longer had to be prepared manually, but could be manufactured on a large scale.

The invention in 1828 of the cocoa press by C. J. Van Houten, a Dutch chocolate master, was revolutionary in terms of helping to cut chocolate prices and bring the product to the mass market. In addition, the cocoa press helped improve the quality of chocolate: by squeezing out some of the cocoa butter (a process known as "dutching"), the beverage's consistency was made much smoother. The onset of the Industrial Revolution helped further, in that as chocolate became mass-produced, its popularity amongst the citizenry spread rapidly.

Nestle's leaflet *The History of Chocolate and Cocoa* documents that from 1800 to the present, the following four factors have been the prime contributors to chocolate's "coming-of-age" as a worldwide food product:

1. the introduction of cocoa powder in 1828;
2. the reduction of excise duties;
3. improvements in transportation facilities, from plantation to factory; and
4. the invention of eating chocolate, and improvements in manufacturing methods.

Credit for the discovery of milk chocolate goes to Daniel Peter of Vevey, Switzerland, who experimented for eight years before finally inventing a means of adding milk to chocolate in 1876. Peter's creation was eventually sold to his neighbor, Henri Nestle, who supplied sweetened condensed milk for the milk chocolate. Today, The Nestle Company, Inc. is the world's largest producer of chocolate.

In 1879 Rodolphe Lindt of Berne, Switzerland, used a procedure called "conching" that helped further refine chocolate to create a product that melted on the tongue. And Swiss confiseur Jules Sechaud of Montreux is credited with introducing a process in 1913 for manufacturing filled chocolates.

Another development of the nineteenth century was the creation of "mole" sauce by some nuns in Puebla, Mexico. Legend has it that the convent was informed it would soon receive a visit from a most important personage of the church. Knowing their stocks were low, the nuns gathered together all they had at hand, killed their only turkey, and concocted a sauce for it that was a blend of chilies, onion, sesame seeds, nuts, and unsweetened chocolate.

CHOCOLATE COMES TO AMERICA

The first time the United States was introduced to bonbons, chocolate creams, hard candies (called "boiled sweets"), and caramels was at Prince Albert's Exposition in 1851 in London. The colonists began by importing their chocolate, but it was understandably expensive to do so, and soon they began to investigate producing their own products.

Chocolate was officially introduced to the United States when John Hannon, an Irish immigrant, brought cocoa beans from the West Indies into Dorchester, Massachusetts, and started milling them. With the financial help of Dr. James Baker, the first chocolate factory in the country was established. The first notice of the sale of cocoa and chocolate in America appeared March 12, 1770, in the Boston *Gazette and Country Journal*:

To be sold by
JOHN BAKER
At his store in Back Street a few Bags of
the best cocoa; also choice Chocolate by
the Hundred or Smaller Quantity.

That enterprise was later to become known for Baker's son, Walter. The business was organized as a corporation in 1895, taking on Liotard's painting of *La Belle Chocolatiere* as its trademark, and remained a family operation until Baker's Chocolate became a division of General Foods in 1927.

Yet part of the real story on chocolate's acceptance by the American colonists dates from the time fishermen from Gloucester, Massachusetts, accepted cocoa beans as payment for cargo in tropical America. Since that time, the product has been recognized as a valuable commodity.

During World War II, the United States government recognized chocolate's importance as a vital source of nourishment, and commissioned Milton S. Hershey to develop a candy bar that the soldiers could carry with them for rations. Another good feature was chocolate's role for "esprit de corps". . . Many a soldier owed his life to a pocket chocolate bar which gave him the strength to carry on until more food rations could be obtained."[23]

The Hershey contribution was repeated again recently, during the Persian Gulf war, when the Pentagon's Defense Personnel Support Center again approached Hershey Foods Corporation to produce a heat-resistant chocolate bar that could withstand temperatures of about 140 degrees. More than 144,000 "Desert Bars" were contracted for a $1.2 million government order, shipped prior to the outbreak of war, and followed by another 750,000 for distribution to the troops once the fighting began.[24] Yet, a "chocolate war" as such broke out in the next bidding contest, and Hershey lost out to M&M/Mars of Hackettstown, New Jersey's "Mars Solid Milk

Chocolate Bar" when its bid of 17.8 cents per bar prevailed over Hershey's 19.2-cent chocolate bar.

In order that cocoa and chocolate buyers and sellers could coordinate their transaction, the New York Cocoa Exchange was established on October 1, 1925, from the original Coffee Exchange. Today the Coffee, Sugar & Cocoa Exchange, located at the World Trade Center, is the world's leading marketplace for futures trading by the 527 membership seats.

THE CURRENT STATE OF CHOCOLATE AROUND THE WORLD

Today, Brazil and the Ivory Coast are leaders in the cocoa bean belt, accounting for nearly half of the world's cocoa (27% and 18% respectively). Africa currently accounts for nearly 60% of all cocoa production, with Ghana only recently being replaced by the Ivory Coast as the most important cocoa-growing country. Total production of cocoa beans globally has remained quite stable for the last two decades, but hit a record level for the 1981-82 crop year of 1.72 million metric tons.

The United States is the world leader in cocoa bean importation, followed by West Germany, the Netherlands, the former U.S.S.R., and the United Kingdom. Together, these countries account for 68% of cocoa imports.

Switzerland continues as the world leader in per capita chocolate consumption. Annual global consumption of cocoa beans averages approximately 600,000 tons, and per capita chocolate consumption is obviously on the rise. It has been said that today we are witnessing a *Chocolate Renaissance*, "a veritable confectionery age of enlightenment"[25] worldwide.

CHOCOLATE FADS, FOLKLORE, AND FANTASIES

Perhaps you're curious about the origins of this book, and about my involvement with chocolate. As you might gather from the Dedication, my mother-in-law was very instrumental in the process of my chocolactivities. For one thing, she certainly passed on her chocolate-oriented genes to my husband, who has withdrawal symptoms if he doesn't have chocolate within a 24-hour period. Yet, heredity has also blended with environment, and, by default, I too have come around to "thinking chocolate."

In 1983, Eric and I were guests of our friends Bill and Emily Mobley[26] at the Media Session for the First International Chocolate Festival, held in New York City. As a social scientist, it struck me that I had never seen so many happy people in the Big Apple. I have never had the opportunity to attend an opium orgy, but the Chocolate Festival had to be the closest thing to it. The participants were smiling and slurping and helping themselves to all the chocolate treats the various chefs had on display. I decided to fudge my way through to finding out what it all meant, this thing called chocolate.

My first move was to construct a marketing survey of chocolate companies around the world–see Appendix A. I contacted nearly 100 chocolate manufacturers and dealers and asked them about the histories of their companies, personnel, sales, advertising, and special features. Some 87 companies responded to my questionnaire: 68 from the United States, four from the Netherlands, three each from Canada and Switzerland, two from Belgium, and one each from Australia, England, France, Ireland, Israel, Mexico, and Puerto Rico. Their answers were reported in a paper entitled "Choco-Marketing-Mania," which was presented in 1985 at the annual meeting of the Popular Culture Association in Louisville, Kentucky. The overwhelming conclusion drawn was that chocolate is a Big Business, one that is and certainly will continue to be marketed with a "consuming passion."

Another result of that study was that I was invited in the spring of 1985 by one of the survey participants, Max Felchlin of Schwyz, Switzerland, to come present my findings on "The State of the Chocolate Industry" to his staff at their factory. Mr. Felchlin also graciously introduced me to other key Swiss people in the chocolate industry, notably Rudy Sprungli; leant me a company car so I could visit the family I had lived with in the French-speaking part of Switzerland as an exchange student; and invited my friend Marilyn Bugg Cooper and me to Max Felchlin Schwyz's fabulous "Vernissage" in Zurich.

Since that visit, I have made it a habit to sample chocolate around the world–Europe (both western and eastern areas), Africa, the Middle East, and Asia. It has been a tough job, but I didn't want to skimp on any resources that might help this chocolate compendium.

Adding to my study, the media for chocolate has also been carefully monitored–see Appendix B. A content analysis was performed on all potential secondary print sources to determine when, where, and how often chocolate was mentioned in the media. In all, 118 magazines, journals, and newspapers have been identified from 1979 to the current day.

This book is the culmination of all that choco-research. It begins, in "Chocolate Fads," discussing the numerous books that have been written on the subject of chocolate: chocolate guides, chocolate cookbooks, chocolate humor, and chocolate specialties. It then discusses chocolate goodies (cakes, candy, cookies, and ice cream), chocolate clubs, chocolate festivals, chocolate fund-raising, chocolate marketing, chocolate media, and more than 100 chocolate novelties. Highlights on the leading chocolate companies are also included in this section.

Although you have already been introduced to chocolate history, you will find many more fascinating chunks of information in "Chocolate Folklore." Studies on chocolate's nutrition are cited, such as its (non)correlation to acne, its tooth decay-inhibiting properties, low caffeine levels (you would have to eat at least a dozen chocolate bars to equal the caffeine amount in one cup of coffee!), caloric and nutritive values, the word on phenylethylamine (the natural substance in the brain reputed to stimulate the same reaction in the body as falling in love!), claims about chocolate's restorative powers and ability to prolong life, and yet, how chocolate can also be lethal to dogs. Other citations include inimitable quotations, including: Milton Hershey at age 85 on his pride in producing the Field Ration D bar for FDR; James Beard on the hot chocolate he drank as a child in Paris; adventurer Henry Savage Landor on using chocolate for his ascent of the Lumpa peaks in the Himalayas; and a letter Thomas Jefferson wrote to John Adams on chocolate's superiority over tea and coffee for health and nourishment. The folklore section also includes chocolate tips and chocolate types and chocolate trivia (do you know which three states allow alcohol in chocolate, when and where the first brownie recipe appeared, who invented the chocolate box, what the best-selling chocolate bar is, where cocoa beans come from, and what is the world's largest chocolate sculpture?) Read on!

"Chocolate Fantasies" starts, appropriately, with chocoholism: the passions, the attitudes, the printing of Madame Chocolate's "Chocolate Creed," a cure one person had for it at the Shick Center for dependence in Los Angeles, chocoholic personality profiles, celebrity confessions, a description of the Type-A consummate chocophile, the obsessions (Arianne Marcus, author of *The Chocolate Bible*, for example, doesn't want to be embalmed, but dipped!), the dieting dilemmas, the ecstacies. Chocolate feasts, chocolate love, chocolate parties, and chocolate promotions are discussed in depth; that is, in deep, dark, chocolatey terms. And finally, chocolate psychology comes into play–for instance, how chocolate has been used as a cure for agoraphobia, a security blanket, an appeal to the senses, a strategy of control, a means to excite passions and curiosities, an excuse gratification, an antidote to guilt, a step toward intimacy, a cause of dependence, a stress-reliever, a restorer of strength, a reward, or maybe just a simple consolation in a world of contracting opportunities.

When you are finished reading *Chocolate Fads, Folklore, and Fantasies,* you can test your chocoknowledge by taking the 200-item Chocoquiz at the end of the book. If your chocoanswers don't tally up well against the chocoquestions, you have several choices: memorize the book so you can beat the odds and reign over your friends at it, and/or eat some chocolate to make you feel better until your next attempt.

The graphics on chocolate ephemera, thanks to William Frost Mobley, should also add to your enjoyment.

For your convenience, some chocolate reference sections are also included: chocolate and chocolate-related companies, and a listing of chocolate resources that have been cited here.

Indisputedly, chocolate is our favorite flavor. It is also, as you are learning, an extremely profitable industry, with many ramifications. You can approach this book from a number of perspectives: for chunks of chocolate knowledge, for fantasy-fulfillment, for a low-cal dive into a forbidden flavor, for a case study of marketing expertise, and/or for pure chocolate enjoyment.

NOTES

1. Linda Corman, *America's Enduring Sweet Tooth*, (February 21, 1993), p. F10.

2. Dudley, Anderson, and Yutzy's *A Study of Chocolate Consumption Among the General Population: A Research Study*, performed in 1984 on 1,003 households in the continental United States on behalf of the Chocolate Manufacturers Association, found that more than eight out of ten households surveyed contained at least one individual who eats desserts, snacks, or drinks beverages made with or containing chocolate.

3. "Let them eat holograms," *New Scientist*, v.130 (April 13, 1991), p.24.

4. Penny Park, "Chocolate checks the chill that kills," *New Scientist*, v.130 (April 20, 1991), p.17.

5. See: Paul Frumkin, "Cookie Chains Cater to Cash-and-Carry Chocoholics." *Nation's Restaurant News*, v.18 (October 15, 1984), p.28.

6. Reported in Adrianne Marcus' *The Chocolate Bible* (Putnam's, 1979). p.28.

7. Frederic and Marcia Morton, *Chocolate: An Illustrated History* (Crown, 1986), p.3.

8. J. S. Fry & Sons, "The Manufacture of Chocolate & Cocoa" (*British Trade Journal*, January 1, 1880), p. 6.

9. See: Walter Baker and Company, *The Chocolate-Plant (Theobroma Cacao) and Its Products* (1891).

10. Cited in Norman Kolpas, *The Chocolate Lover's Companion* (Quick Fox, 1977), p. 128.

11. Ambrosia Chocolate Company of Milwaukee points out in its book *The Story of Cacao: "Food of the Gods"* (1945) that "Since the Greek gods who lived on Mt. Olympus were said to have lived on a food called 'ambrosia,' the meaning of the word 'Theobroma' can be roughly translated into English by the word 'ambrosia.'"

12. Walter Baker & Co., *The Chocolate-Plant*, 1891.

13. Fernando Alvarez de Toledo, 1508-1582.

14. Cited in Adrianne Marcus, *The Chocolate Bible* (Putnam's, 1979), p. 27-8.

15. Walter Baker & Co., *Cocoa and Chocolate Exhibits* (Barta Press, 1915), p.17.

16. 1791-1834.

17. Repeated in Carol Ann Rinzler's *The Book of Chocolate* (St. Martin's Press, 1977), pp. 128-9.

18. J. S. Fry & Sons, "The Manufacturer of Chocolate & Cocoa" (*British Trade Journal*, January 1, 1880). p.3.

19. Chocosuisse, the Union of Swiss Chocolate Manufacturers' *Chocologie*, p.6.

20. Ibid.

21. B. P. Forbes, *Chocolate and Cocoa* (Cleveland, 1903). p.6.

22. Joseph H. Fries, "Chocolate: A Review of Published Reports of Allergic and Other Deleterious Effects Real or Presumed," *Annals of Allergy,* v.41, #4 (October 1978). p.1.

23. The Chocolate Manufacturers Association of the U.S.A.'s *The Story of Chocolate* (1960). p.8.

24. Source: Bonnie L. Glass. public relations representative for the Hershey Foods Corporation, Hershey, PA.

25. Lesly Berger, *The Gourmet's Guide to Chocolate* (New York: Quill, 1984), p. 9.

26. Bill, who has written the Foreword to *Chocolate Fads, Folklore, and Fantasies,* owns a priceless collection of chocolate ephemera. Articles on it have appeared in both *Smithsonian* (Ruth Mehrtens Galvin, 1986) and *Americana* (Gayle Turim, 1990).

Chapter II

Chocolate Fads

CHOCOLATE BOOKS

- The **first book** completely devoted to the subject of chocolate was Cardenas' *Libro en el cual trata del chocolate*, published in Mexico in 1609. Then, in 1624, Joan Franc Rauch wrote "Disputatio Medico Dioetetica de Aere et Esculentis, de Necnon Potu," a condemnation of cocoa as a violent inflamer of the passions. In 1631 Colmenero's *A Curious Treatise of the Nature of Chocolate* was published in Madrid; it became the standard work of the century, translated into many languages and passing through a series of editions.

- **Walter Baker Company**, which established the first chocolate factory in the United States in 1765, produced several publications, including:
  1. *The Chocolate-Plant (Theobroma Cacao) and Its Products*, 891.
  2. *Cocoa and Chocolate: A Short History of Their Production and Use*, 1910.
  3. *Cocoa and Chocolate Exhibits*, 1915.

- *The Chocolate Book* is a **children's book** with recipes, chocolate lore, poems, and yummy illustrations–available from Caedmon Publishers.

- Other **children's chocolate books** include these:
  1. *Chocolate Marshmelephant Sundae* by cartoonist Mike Thaler (Franklin Watts, 1978) is a delightful collection of "tickletoons," jokes, riddles, and puns.

2. Pre-teens will enjoy Robert Kimmel Smith's *Chocolate Fever* (Dell, 1972). It begins, "There are some people who say that Henry Green wasn't really born, but was hatched, fully grown, from a chocolate bean." Henry loved and needed chocolate in his diet; he loved and needed chocolate "bittersweet, light, dark, and daily." That is, until the day he broke out with chocolate fever, when he began to smell like chocolate and to taste like chocolate . . .

3. *The Chocolate Wars* by Robert Cormier (Dell, 1974) chronicles what happens to a high-schooler who decides not to participate in the all-school fund-raising project of selling chocolate bars.

- *Chocolate Artistry* by Elaine Gonzalez (Contemporary, 1984) contains information on techniques for molding, decorating, and designing with chocolate.

- *The Chocolate Bible* (G.P. Putnam, 1979) chronicles Adrianne Marcus' guide to the best chocolates in the United States, Canada, and Europe.

- Sandra Boynton's *Chocolate, The Consuming Passion* (Workman, 1982) contains irresistible cartoons describing many facets of our relationships with chocolate. The book sold 600,000 copies in the United States, and more than 100,000 in the United Kingdom.

- Pauline G. Child's *The "Exclusively Chocolate" Cookbook* (PGC Publications, 1984) incorporates **convenience** foods into its recipes.

- In an attempt to answer the chocolate-lover's dreams, *Betty Crocker* released its *Chocolate Cookbook* (Random House, 1985), billed as "a sublime celebration of chocolate indulgence in all its infinite variety."

- Mary Jane Finsand's *The Diabetic Chocolate Cookbook* (Sterling, 1984) calls for carob, a chocolate substitute. One tablespoon of carob has the same calorie count as one tablespoon of cocoa.

- In her **Book of Divine Indulgences** (Contemporary Books, 1983), Elaine Sherman, known as "Madame Chocolate," proclaims chocolate as "heavenly, milky, sensual, deep, dark, sumptuous, gratifying, potent, dense, creamy, seductive, suggestive, rich, excessive, silky, smooth, luxurious, celestial." More than 100 recipes include "tips on selecting, tempering, serving, storing and decorating with chocolate. From Swiss to Belgian to American; from unsweetened to bittersweet to semi-sweet; from milk chocolate to white chocolate to gianduja; from chips to chunks to morsels and drops. Chocolate is explored in its infinite varieties."

- When the food editors of **Farm Journal Magazine** asked readers to send in their favorite chocolate recipes, they received an unprecedented 10,000 entries in two weeks. The 275 cakes, cookies, candies, brownies, pies, mousses, sauces, and fudge judged the best are included in Elise W. Manning's *Farm Journal's Choice Chocolate Recipes* (Ballantine, 1978).

- Lesly Berger's **The Gourmet's Guide to Chocolate** (Quill, 1984) reviews the chocolates that represent the "creme de la creme of chocolate" from more than a dozen nations.

- Lora Brody's **Growing Up on the Chocolate Diet** (Little, Brown, 1985) is a combination cookbook/memoir with advice on how to maintain chocolate as a healthy passion.

- In celebration of its 50th anniversary, the Hershey Chocolate Company reissued its **Hershey's 1934 Cookbook**. The revised edition plays on a nostalgic theme of how chocolate has remained an all-American favorite.

- In 1892 Richard Cadbury put together a volume entitled *Cocoa: All About It*. Cited as authored by **"Historicus,"** it is packed with curious old quotations about the product.

- To keep you from having to poke your finger into every chocolate, Hal and Ellen Greenberg have written **Inside Chocolate: The Chocolate Lover's Guide to Boxed Chocolate** (Harry N.

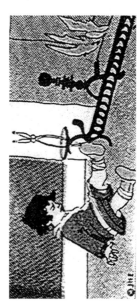

THE CHOCOLATE MAN

In Bon Bon Town once on a time ◈ Lived Dan, the hero of this rhyme; ◈ And his thoughts on candy so often ran ◈ That his folks all called him Sweet Tooth Dan; ◈ Every time Dan got a cent ◈ In the candy shop 'twould soon be spent; ◈ He ate so many caramel creams ◈ That they followed him into the Land o'Dreams ◈ So, napping one day, young

Sweet Tooth Dan ◈ Dreamed the dream of the Chocolate Man.

The Chocolate Man on a store shelf stood ◈ And pointed a gun at a candy wood ◈ Where a candy bird with candy wings ◈ Flew over all kinds of candy things, ◈ A-singing a candy song so sweet ◈ That powdered sugar soon covered its feet ◈ And filled the air with candied tunes ◈ That rose and fell like toy balloons ◈ Till they burst on the ear of Sweet Tooth Dan ◈ And he looked in and spied that Chocolate Man.

Dan dreamed that he from his home had come ◈ Clutching a dime 'twixt finger and thumb ◈ To buy for Mother a birthday gift ◈ And run back home so very swift ◈ He'd never be missed until

Abrams, 1985). In 26 luscious full-color "portraits," various chocolates are identified.

- John and Marilyn Cooper, who own "Sweet Daddy's" in Wayne, Pennsylvania, consider Nancy Baggett's *The International Chocolate Cookbook* (Stewart, Tabori & Chang, 1991) the best book of the bunch.

- Martine **Jolly**, a well-known French cook, has written a book touted as "really haute" cuisine: *Le Chocolat* (Pantheon, 1985).

- Judith Olney's *Joy of Chocolate* (Barron, 1982) includes some nontraditional uses for chocolate, such as pate, strawberry short-cake, crepes, terrain, and a white chocolate quiche. This volume is also available on videocassettes.

- Sylvia Balser Hirsch, the celebrated **"Miss Grimble,"** has written a delightful collection of recipes in *Chocolate Crazy* (Macmillan, 1984).

- **"50 Years Pralinosa"** is a handsome booklet produced in 1985 by Max Felchlin of Schwyz, Switzerland, in commemoration of the company's continuing commitment to quality chocolate. The brochure features pictures of glazes, cakes, pastries, cookies, and tea cakes made with Felchlin's pralinosa.

- Ruth Moorman and Lalla Williams' *The Seven Chocolate Sins* (Quail Ridge Press, 1979) contains more than 200 chocolate recipes dedicated to the notion that anything as good as chocolate must be immoral.

- *Sweet Seduction: Chocolate Truffles* (Harper Colophon, 1984) by Adrienne Welch offers both beautiful photos and practical advice on making special confections.

- Pam Williams of Au Chocolat in Vancouver, British Columbia, has put together more than six dozen recipes from her many years of **"truffletiering"** in *Oh Truffles* (Wilmor, 1983).

(Note: Consider this–we have had chocolate books for nearly four centuries! Dozens more chocolate books and publications are cited throughout this book. Their growing numbers are just one more indication of the developing chocolate phenomenon.)

CHOCOLATE GOODIES

Cakes

- Once the zucchini and fruits of summer are no longer available for chocolate creations, **autumn** encourages additions like pumpkin and cranberries to chocolate cakes. As the holidays arrive, you might want to make chocolate gingerbread men.

- **"Baumkuchen,"** literally means "Tree Cake"–it is a fine Old World cake baked on a rotisserie, then layered in dark or white chocolate. Weighing about 3 lbs, the 12″ King of Cakes is available at Stork's Pastry Shop in Whitestone, NY.

- The favorite chocolate cake of the Swiss has been declared to be "Schwarzwaldertorte," **Black Forest Cake.**

- **Boston Cream Pie**, a custard-filled and chocolate-covered sponge cake, was first served at Boston's Parker House Hotel in 1856.

- Folklore has it that **brownies** evolved around the 1920s as a mistake. "Brownies are the classic comfort food, the perfect compensation for a busy life," according to Leslie Land, author of *The New England Epicure*. By definition, she contends, there is not such thing as a pretentious brownie.

- The critical evaluation in **brownie-making**, according to Linda Burum, author of *Brownies* (Scribner's, 1984), is texture–which is affected by ratios of ingredients.

- There are a number of **cake fillings** that blend beautifully with chocolate, including: mocha/coffee, vanilla, almond, rum, peppermint, cherry, orange, brandy, and various fruit preserves.

- Evan's of Topeka, Kansas, offers its recipe for a chocolate-filled, liqueur-laced **cheesecake** for $2.

- Rosie's of Boston has developed an award-winning fudgy brownie called **"Chocolate Orgasm."** It was voted "Best Brownie" by *Boston Magazine* from 1980-84 and "Best Brownie in America" in C. Paul Wongo's "America's Best 100." More than 5,000 brownies are sold at Rosie's each week.

- The late James Beard has labeled the **Chocolate Velvet Cake** at the Four Seasons Restaurant in New York City "that delectable super-mousse which combines eggs, butter, and chocolate to make the greatest chocolate dessert I have ever tasted."

- "In my opinion, as well as that of practically everyone else, there is no more fitting **crown to a festive occasion** than a chocolate cake. By that I mean an honest chocolate cake–be it Fudge Layer Cake, Marble Chiffon, Red Devil's Food, or what-you-will. I mean a cake built from the finest ingredients: dark rich chocolate, fresh country eggs, sweet cream butter, mixed with loving care and a dash of eager anticipation."

  –Gertrude Parke, *The Big Chocolate Cookbook*
  (A & W Visual Library, 1968, p. 30)

- The Swiss Colony of Monroe, Wisconsin, are creators of the original chocolate **"Dobosh Torte,"** eight layers of chocolate-filled and coated cake, available in four different sizes. It's also available in double chocolate!

- *Farm Journal's Choice Chocolate Recipes* (Ballantine Books, 1978) contains cake recipes for Whole Wheat Chocolate Cake, Zucchini Chocolate Cake, Red Beet Chocolate Cake, Chocolate Sauerkraut Cake, Egyptian Chocolate Cake, Chocolate/Lemon Layer Cake, Delightful Apricot/Fudge Cake, Chocolate/Vinegar Cake, Pumpkin Chocolate Cake, and Pineapple Chocolate Cupcakes.

- When **French Silk Chocolate Pie** was first introduced in a bake-off contest in 1951, it won the $1,000 first prize.

- Cafe Beaujolais Bakery in Mendocino, California, offers a 20-oz **chocolate fruitcake** made with dried fruit and bittersweet chocolate.

- **Mable Hoffman's** *Chocolate Cookery* (Dell, 1978) contains these intriguing recipes for chocolate cakes: Mississippi Mud, Banana-Nut, Peachy Cream, Peanut Butter Streusel, Date, Chocolate Fruitcake, and Chocolate Chip Chiffon.

- Of the several thousand members representing 28 countries who belong to the International Cake Exploration Society **(ICES)**, Marge Kehoe of Springfield, Massachusetts, was the first to introduce an iced chocolate cake.

- **Maison Glass** in New York City offers David Glass' incomparable cakes, such as his chocolate mousse cake, through mail order.

- Let Them Eat Cake, out of Eugene, Oregon, offers various chocolate **cake mixes**, such as Moist Mocha Orange and Rich Chocolate Buttermilk.

- Rose Beranbaum's *Romantic and Classic Cakes* (Irene Chalmers, 1981) is considered the definitive guide to cooking with chocolate. Beranbaum is the creator of the best thermometer for tempering chocolate.

- Every day the Hotel Sacher in Vienna fills about two- to three-hundred mail order requests for its famous **Sacher Torte**, first concocted in 1832 by Franz Sacher when he was an apprentice in the court of Prince Clemens von Metternich.

- Martin Johner, "The Chocolate Chef," of the Culinary Center of New York, has superseded his chocolate fettucini invention with **chocolate sushi**, wafer-thin chocolate crepes with chocolate filling made from creme fraiche that are dipped in dark chocolate sauce.

- Harry & David offer a 9-layer, 3-3/4-lb **chocolate torte** that serves 20 people, plus a 2-lb French chocolate cheesecake, out of their Medford, Oregon, store.

- Norm Thompson of Portland, Oregon, fills lots of mail orders for his famous **Truffle Cake**.

- In her *Ultimate Chocolate Cake Book* (Holt, Rinehart, & Winston, 1984), Pam Asquith doesn't use any chemical leaveners; rather, she offers melted chocolate as a base, bound with ground nuts or flour and leavened with beaten eggs or egg whites.

- *Wild About Brownies* by Barbara Albright and Leslie Wiener (Barron, 1985) suggests some wild brownie variations.

Candy

- **Baby Ruth** candy bars are not named for the famous "Home Run King" baseball player, but for President Grover Cleveland's youngest daughter, Ruth.

- Perugina's **"Baci,"** the company's best-known candy, is the Italian word for "kisses."

- The Nestle Company, Inc. accounts for about 60% of the **boxed chocolate** in the United States. As such, it conducts frequent market research studies of boxed chocolate, and in 1983 found a 50% increase in six years. Seven out of ten Americans interviewed reported 3.2 purchases per year, nearly half at specialty candy stores for "luxury" chocolates.

- Alison and Margaret Engels, authors of *Food Finds*, judge **Brigittine Fudge** the best ever tasted; it's made by the Brigittine Monks of Woodside, California.

- According to the National Confectioners Association, National Candy Wholesalers Association, and Retail Confectioners International, here are **caloric** listings of some of your favorite brand items:

Product	Serving Size	Calories
Almond Joy	1.6 oz	220
Baby Ruth	2.28	320
Butterfinger	2.16	290
Charleston Chew	1.87	220
5th Avenue	1.75	249
Goo Goo Cluster	1.75	245
Heath Bars	1.16	150
Hershey's Milk Choc.	1.45	220
Junior Mints	1.6	190
Kit Kat	1.5	210
Krackel	1.45	220
M&Ms Peanut	1.67	240
M&Ms Plain	1.69	240
Mars Bar	1.87	260
Milky Way Bar	2.1	270
Mr. Goodbar	1.65	270
Nestle $100,000	1.5	200
Nestle Crunch	1.06	160
Pom Poms	1.58	190
Reese's PB Cups (2)	1.6	240
Snickers Bar	2.0	270
3 Musketeers	2.28	280
York Peppermint Pattie	1.5	180

- Ronsvalles of Syracuse, New York, is famous for its **"Chippies,"** chocolate patties with little pieces of potato chips in them. They also make "Chippie-bars."

- You can still get **Chocolate Babies** at the "Penny Candy" counter of the (Manchester Center) Vermont Country Store.

- The **"chocolate bar"** was discovered in the nineteenth century when chemists found they could extract the fat from cocoa beans and mix the resultant cocoa butter with sugar into a thin paste, then mold it into bar-like shapes. Daniel Peter of Switzerland is credited with perfecting a solid milk chocolate for eating in 1875.

- A **"Chocolot Candy Maker"** for children can be ordered through Grandma's House in Wetumpka, Alabama.

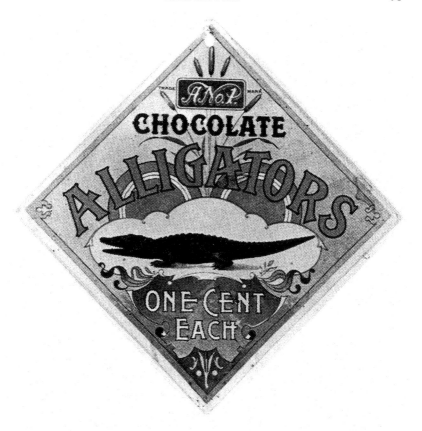

- Nestle, which introduced **chocolate chips** in 1939, today produces about 250 million of them each day. There are approximately 675 chocolate chip morsels in each 12-oz bag.

- For more than a century, Cella's Confections, Inc. of New York has been the only chocolate manufacturer in the country to make **chocolate-covered cherries** with a liquid center. Each package contains this message: "Chocolate-Covered Cherries with 100% Liquid Center."

- Ray Broekel has written *The Chocolate Chronicles* (Wallace-Homestead, 1985), a history of how various nickel candy bars

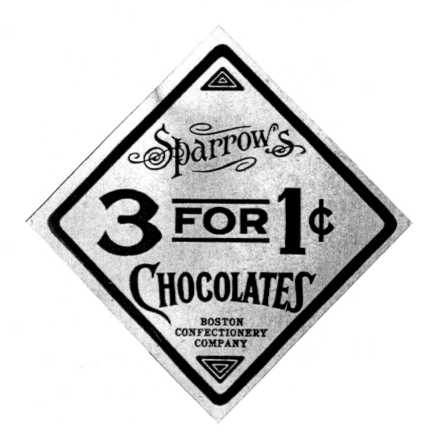

were developed and named, and how they add to our chocolate heritage.

- **Fudge** was popular in the early 1900s at northeastern women's colleges. *The American Heritage Cookbook* (American Heritage Publishing, 1964) reports that often it was cooked over gaslight as an excuse for parties after "lights-out." While the standard formula was "3-2-1" (3 squares chocolate, 2 cups sugar, 1 cup cream), Smith students included granulated as well as brown sugar and molasses; Vassarites used less chocolate and butter; and Wellesley women are credited with adding marshmallows to the cooked fudge.

- Maynards of London makes a **chocolate ginger** candy of pure Australian ginger covered with chocolate.

- More than 150,000 **Goo Goo Clusters**–a candy made up of chocolate, peanuts, caramel, and marshmallows–are produced each day by Standard Candy Company of Nashville, Tennessee.

- The complete recipe for the "original" **Heath Bar** has remained a company secret for more than 80 years.

- **Hershey's Kisses**, first made in 1907, are produced today at the rate of approximately 20-25 million per day. Each kiss is wrapped in five square inches of foil wrap, and contains 25 calories.

- Peggy Mellody and Linda Rosenbloom have written *In the Chips* (Rawson, 1985), which they call the first complete chocolate chip cookbook. The 216 recipes plus variations include breads, cakes, candies, desserts, cookies, sauces, ice creams, beverages, and garnishes.

- According to Mars, Inc. of Hackettstown, New Jersey, **M&M** stands for "Mars and Murrie," the company's founders. A bowl of 100 M&Ms breaks down to these color combinations: 40 brown, 20 yellow, 20 orange, 10 green, and 10 tan. The red M&Ms were discontinued in 1976 because of the health controversy surrounding the use of red dye.

- **M&M/Mars** is a $1.4 billion business, with 43% of the chocolate bar market. (Snickers alone accounts for $300 million.) Hershey bars claim another 24% of the industry, while Peter Paul Cadbury has only 8%. Together, M&M/Mars and Hershey manufacture all of the ten best-selling candy bars–and most of the top 20.

- Master pastry chef Albert Kumin, one of the founders of the International Pastry Arts Center, offers directions for a **chocolate nativity** scene in the January 1990 issue of *Chocolatier.*

- **Nestle's** 10-lb chocolate bars, which it sells to chocolate candy makers and industrial users, all bear the name of the founder of milk chocolate: Daniel Peter of Vevey, Switzerland. The company's latest introduction to the market is its "Alpine White with Almonds," billed as a European-style "white chocolate" specialty.

- **O'Henry Bars** don't derive from O. Henry (pseudonym for the writer William Sydney Porter), but in honor of a strong young man who worked at George Williamson's candy factory. The story was that when the women workers couldn't move the heavy barrels of corn syrup, they would call, "Oh, Henry!"

- A milk chocolate **orange**, shaped like a real orange and divided into 20 pieces, is made by Joseph Terry & Sons, Ltd. of the United Kingdom from a combination of milk chocolate and orange oil.

- **"Orange Milk Chocolate Crunch,"** made by Harvey Merckens and distributed by Florida Chocolate Specialties, contains a "Greetings from Florida" sign on each chocolate bar.

- You can get "Candy by the Yard," a 3-foot, 3-lb assortment, from **Price's Fine Chocolates** of Kansas City, Missouri.

- **Raisinets**, chocolate-covered raisins, are the best-selling candy at theatre candy counters.

- They're only available in July, but you've never had anything like chocolate-covered Oregon **raspberries**, available through Karl Bissinger of St. Louis, Missouri.

- Munson's Candy Kitchen in Bolton, Connecticut, offers chocolate-dipped **strawberries** from Father's Day through Fourth of July weekend.

- The #1 selling candy bar in the United States is **Snickers**. According to the National Candy Buyers Brands Survey, it is the all-American favorite.

- Bendicks of Mayfair, a British chocolate company that has been awarded the Royal Warrant, has a **"Sporting and Military Chocolate"** bittersweet candy bar.

- The original **3 Musketeers Bar** of 1932 had three parts–chocolate, vanilla, and strawberry. In the 1940s it became all chocolate.

- Tobler-Suchard's most famous product is its **"Toblerone"** candy bar, shaped like the Swiss Alps. It was first developed in 1908 by Theodor Tobler and his cousin Emil Baumann, and sells today in over 100 countries. A wrapper announcing Toblerone as "the first patented Swiss milk chocolate" was used from 1920-31; later it was changed to indicate that Toblerone is "Swiss milk chocolate with almond and honey nougat."

- **Tootsie Rolls** were named in 1896 by inventor Leo Hirschfield in honor of his daughter. The first wrapped penny candy, Tootsie Roll sales for 1984 were $93 million.

- At the San Francisco Chocolate Company you can get a **"Truffwich,"** two slim wafers filled with ganache, then dipped in chocolate; it resembles a sandwich.

- American candy-makers are **upgrading** old chocolate bars–like Hershey's new "Big Block," or Peter Paul Cadbury's "Thick Bar."

- **"Wilbur Buds"** look like–but actually predate–Hershey's Kisses; the Wilbur Chocolate Company dates back to 1884.

- At Alethea's in Buffalo, New York, you can get **yogurt chocolate** candy. They also have exotic chocolate-covered Chinese ginger fruit candies.

- While Hershey Food Corporation and M&M/Mars still dominate the **U.S. candy market**, Switzerland's Nestle, Britain's Cadbury Schweppes, and Finland's Huhtamaki (which bought Good & Plenty, Clark Bars, and Milk Duds in 1983) are emerging as formidable competitors.

- The first **Whitman Sampler** appeared in 1912, unique not only for its old-fashioned design but its index to where chocolates could be located. To this day, it still accounts for a sizeable portion of the $100 million company.

Cookies

- Chocolate cookies used for **baking** are usually one of three types:

1. Chocolate snap–like a ginger snap in size and shape, it is easy to crush and use in combination with other ingredients
2. Chocolate wafer–a flat, thin, dark and colored cookie that can be crushed or served with whipped cream between its layers
3. Frosting-filled chocolate cookies–brand names like Oreo or Hydrox (the debate rages on!), these are especially good crushed up for pie crusts or "smooshed" into ice cream

- **Brownies** began around 1914. Famous chocolate dessert expert Maida Heatter has claimed they owe their origin to "Brownie" Schrumpf, an octogenarian food authority from Bangor, Maine.

- If you want to "Say It with Chocolate," **Cookie Bloomers** of Connecticut (800/437-SEND) ships cookie arrangements anywhere in the country.

- Nestle reports that home bakers make more than seven billion **chocolate chip cookies** per year with their Toll House Morsels.

- **Chocolate chip cookie sales** add up to more than $7 billion annually.

- *Consumer Reports* (February 1985) tested more than two dozen popular brands of the more than 140 varieties of chocolate chip cookies, plus several cookie mixes and four boutique/fresh-baked types (Mrs. Fields, Grand Union, David's, and Famous Amos). Three brands stood out as excellent in terms of "total chocolate impact and chip texture": the bake-it-yourself Duncan Hines mix, Mrs. Fields, and store-baked Grand Union cookies. The overall loser was Murray, which "seemed to contain no chips; instead, the cookies sported meager chocolate smears almost totally lacking in chocolate character."

- Burnham & Brady, Inc. in East Hartford, Connecticut, feature the **"Cookie Chip Chocolate"**–a reverse chocolate chip cookie of chocolate stuffed with bits of cookie.

- First to recognize the possibilities of designer-baked goods, Wally Amos (with Leroy Robinson) tells the story of his company's development about ten years ago in *The Famous Amos Story: The Face That Launched a Thousand Chips* (Doubleday, 1983).

- From recipes that won a National Chocolate Chip Cookie Contest, Larry and Honey Zisman have compiled *The 47 Best Chocolate Chip Cookies in the World* (St. Martin's Press, 1983).

- Chocolate Emotions of Sunnyside, New York, sells a dozen **Guilty Bars,** loaded with chocolate chips and pecans and a warning label: "This dessert may destroy your ability to be crabby and can cause you to smile for no apparent reason . . ."

- Sunshine Biscuits introduced **Hydrox Cookies** in 1908, naming them for a combination of hydrogen and oxygen as symbols of purity and cleanliness. Nabisco brought out rival Oreo cookies in 1912.

- Pepperidge Farm offers a 12″, 1-1/2-lb **mail-order chocolate chip cookie.**

- If you want to set up your own **chocolate chip cookie operation,** contact the American Enterprise Association in Los Angeles for their instruction manual.

- Last year, Americans spent $2.5 billion for cookies, more than $200 million for fresh-baked, soft-and-chewy, **over-the-counter** ones. Some of the best known include those made by the Original Great American Chocolate Cookie Company, Famous Amos, Mrs. Fields, David's, Unknown Jerome, Famous Chocolate Cookie Company, Cooky Wooky, Le Dernier Chip, Tom's Mom's, and The Original Cookie Company. It is predicted that the market for over-the-counter cookies will double next year.

- According to Nabisco, which makes moist-and-chewy "Almost Home" cookies, more than 200 million pounds of **packaged chocolate chip cookies** are sold each year. Other competition includes: Keebler's "Soft Batch" (soft inside, crunchy outside), Frito Lay's "Grandma's Rich 'n Chewy" (crispy outside, chewy in), and Proctor and Gamble's "Duncan Hines Chocolate Chip Cookies" (chewy inside, crispy out).

- **Sweet Victory** in New York markets its chocolate chip cookies as lower than others in calories, cholesterol, and fat.

- Chocolate chip cookies were first introduced by Ruth Wakefield in 1931 at the **Toll House** Restaurant in Whitman, Massachusetts, when she chopped up a semisweet chocolate bar and put it into a batch of cookie dough. She later sold the rights to the Nestle Company, who have (wisely) perpetuated "Toll House Cookies."

- Throughout World War II, **Ruth Wakefield** sent Toll House cookies to American servicemen all around the world.

Ice Cream

- Known for its ice cream-dipping stores throughout New Hampshire, Weeks has an especially exciting concoction in its **Almond Joy,** combining fresh coconut and its extract with chocolate-covered almonds.

- Loving Spoonful gets raves from lots of University of Michigan students who go to the Ann Arbor Ice Cream shop for **Bailey's Irish Cream**.

- **Banana Fudge**–from Berkeley, California. McCallum's, a family-owned business for half a century, makes this ice cream from its own homemade fudge and fresh bananas.

- **Ben and Jerry's**, the Burlington, Vermont-based ice cream manufacturers who brought you Dastardly Mash, Oreo Mint, and Heath Bar amongst other chocolate favorites, is a multimillion-dollar business.

- Ashley's of New Haven, Connecticut, named for the world-champion Frisbee-catching dog Ashley Whippet, has a legendary

bittersweet chocolate ice cream that blends pure chocolate chips into a chocolate liquor base.

- With a commitment to quality and natural ingredients since it started in Philadelphia in 1866, **Breyers'** Mint Chocolate Chip is available in supermarkets from the Atlantic to the Mississippi River.

- To make its **cherry chocolate chip** ice cream, the Mayfield Dairy in Athens, Tennessee, uses the "shatter method," whereby liquid chocolate is poured into the freezing mix, coming out as oddly shaped chocolate chunks.

- A Boston favorite since 1914, **Brigham's** has ice cream specialties like Boston Cream Pie, Irish Coffee, and Mocha Almond.

- **Chipwich**, a sandwich made of ice cream between two chocolate chip cookies, was invented by Richard LaMotta of Brooklyn. The discovery has made him a millionaire.

- At Gorton's in Fresno, California, you can sample **Chocolate Alaskan Chip**, a dark chocolate ice cream sprinkled with white chocolate mint chips.

- Bailey's has been a famous Boston confectionary landmark and ice cream emporium since 1900–especially prized for its **chocolate chip** ice cream that's made from Bailey's own shaved pure chocolate candy mixed into rich vanilla ice cream.

- One of the trademarks of New York City's **Chocolate Garden** at 1390 Third Avenue is its "stuffed" ice cream–the flavor of your choice stuffed with butter crunch, nonpareils, chocolate peanuts, and/or smashed malt balls.

- You've never given **chocolate ice** a chance until you've tasted the combination of shaved ice, cocoa, and fudge at the Caffe Roma, located in New York's Little Italy since 1891.

- Steve's Homemade, winner of two local awards for the best ice cream in Atlanta, has developed an unusual **cinnamon chocolate chip** ice cream.

- Ice cream **cones** are dipped in white chocolate before being filled at Le Chocolatier in Latham, New York.

- *Consumer Reports* (July 1986) gave these four brands of chocolate ice cream the highest ratings for flavor and texture: Baskin Robbins, Ben and Jerry's, Breyers, and Friendly's.

- Graeter's of Cincinnati has made its **Double Chocolate Chip** ice cream the same way since 1870: with its own chocolate candies churned and whipped up by an ice cream paddle.

- **DoveBar** International, Inc. of Northfield, Illinois, has recently introduced a hand-dipped chocolate-flavored ice cream bar; the flavors are vanilla, chocolate, coffee, and strawberry.

- **"Eskimo Pie"** was patented January 24, 1922, by Christian Nelson of Iowa.

- Marshall Fields of Chicago is famous for its **Frango Mint** ice cream, made from its own mint-flavored chocolate.

- My town of Wilbraham, Massachusetts, is best known as headquarters to **Friendly's,** a local ice cream tradition begun in 1935. They have many chocolate offerings, but my personal favorite continues to be its Swiss Chocolate Almond Sundae.

- Serendipity, located in Boston's Faneuil Hall Marketplace, serves **Frozen Hot Chocolate**, a concoction of 12 different imported chocolates that is a cross between a frappe and a chocolate sherbet.

- Dean of Italian chocolatiers since 1860, Pernigotti produces a scrumptious chocolate **gelato.**

- Originally a dairy business in Minnesota in 1882, Bridgeman's was acquired by Land O' Lakes in 1952. Its **German Chocolate** ice cream is 2/3 chocolate, 1/3 caramel, coconut, and German chocolate syrup.

- Snelgrove, located in Salt Lake City, Utah, since 1929, now has ice cream flavors like its **German Chocolate Cake** available in grocery stores, hotels, and local ice cream parlors.

- **Gialduia gelato**, a combination of chocolate ice cream and hazelnuts, is an Italian tradition carried on at Procopio Gelateria in Seattle.

- Lickety Split, located in New York's East Village, mixes different cookie combinations into its ice cream, the best being its chocolate **Girl Scout** varieties.

- **Haagen-Daz**, the Danish-sounding ice cream emporium headquartered in Westwood, New Jersey, is indisputably the largest purveyor of super-premium ice cream in the country. Have you ever tried their chocolate chocolate chip?

- Bailey's of Boston is credited with being the inventor of the **hot fudge sundae**. The 100+-year-old company has 8 stores, and has multimillion-dollar annual sales.

- You can get ambrosia ice cream like French Double Chocolate, Chocolate Showers, Chocolate Amaretto, or Chocolate Grand Marnier at **Liled's** Candy Kitchen in Vallejo, California.

- In true Italian style, try **Martinica** (chocolate rum) ice cream at Marco's Gelato d'Italia in Eugene, Oregon.

- Polar Bear Ice Cream of Santa Cruz runs an annual "fantasy flavor" contest, and can thank one of its winners for **Mexican Chocolate**, a dark chocolate ice cream flavored with chocolate chips, almonds, cinnamon, spices, and a dash of lemon rind.

- **Montezuma** has been credited with being the "Father of Chocolate Ice Cream"; he reportedly took snow from a volcano and poured whipped, frothy "chocolatl" over it in the early sixteenth century.

- The Chocolate Shop, a Kalamazoo, Michigan, landmark since 1917, has a notable **Nesselrode** ice cream made from a chocolate base with rum, raisins, nuts, and candy fruit.

- Emack and Bolio's of Boston was the first company to introduce **Oreo Cookies** ice cream.

- Buckman's Ice Cream Village, a Rochester, New York, tradition since 1911, has developed its own **Oreo Speedwagon**.

- If you like the combination, you'll rave over Kimball Farm's **Peanut Butter Chocolate Chip**. The three-generation business, located in Westford, Massachusetts, also has a memorable Mint Oreo.

- At the Via Dolce Confectioners in Venice, California, you can get remarkable **Raspberry Chocolate Truffle** ice cream, featuring Pacific Northwest black raspberries.

- Dreyer's Grand Ice Cream Company, founded in Oakland in 1928, invented **Rocky Road** ice cream.

- **Sanders**, a Detroit operation since 1875, is credited with inventing the ice cream soda. It makes its chocolate chip ice cream with ground toffee coated in chocolate.

- Herrell's in Northampton, Massachusetts, carries on Steve Herrell's innovation of the **"Smoosh-In!,"** where bits of M&Ms, Junior Mints, Reese's Peanut Butter Cups, Heath Bars, Oreos, and Mounds are "smooshed" into your favorite (chocolate?!) ice cream.

- The Ice Cream Works in Denver has brought to ice cream that old camping favorite of graham crackers, marshmallows, and chocolate: **S'mores**.

- **Barbra Streisand's** favorite snack is coffee ice cream with chocolate fudge sauce–the kind that hardens when it hits the ice cream.

- When **Stroh's Brewery**, which was founded in Detroit in 1850, decided to diversify during the Prohibition era, it began an ice cream business. Formulas developed more than 60 years ago are still used as the basis for its flavors, including Chocolate Almond, Rocky Road, and Chocolate Marshmallow recipes.

- **Thomas Sweet** keeps Princeton University students happy with its Oreos and Cream, Chocolate Mousse, and Chocolate Chip Cookie ice cream.

- In 1948, **Swenson's** opened its first shop in San Francisco; today it has more than 300 ice creameries, featuring such delights as Sticky Chewy Chocolate, Caramel Turtle Fudge, and Swiss Orange Chip.

- Giffords of Silver Spring, Maryland, began in 1938, and today continues its tradition of such favorites as **Swiss Chocolate** ice cream, which is made with Gifford's own chocolate candy.

- Goodnoe's of Newtown, Pennsylvania, a dairy tradition there since 1918, won the National Ice Cream Retailers Association's certificate of merit for its **Swiss Chocolate Almond** ice cream.

- **"Tre Scalini"** chocolate ice cream at Neal's in Houston was chosen as "the nation's most resplendent" in Carol T. Robbins and Herbert Wolff's *The Very Best: ICE CREAM and Where to Find It* (The Very Best: Publishers, Inc., 1982). Instead of cocoa, this chocolate ice cream is made of 30% pre-processed chocolate liquor.

- Dreyer's Grand Ice Cream Company is the parent company of the newly developed **Tres Chocolate**, which features these flavors: Chocolate Decadence, Chocolate Chocolate Chunk, Chocolate Cappuccino, Chocolate Hazelnut Fudge, Chocolate Almond Chocolate, Chocolate Raspberry, Milk Chocolate, and Chocolate Toasted Almond.

- If you like them as candies, you'll flip over **Turtles** as ice cream—especially at Petersen's Ice Cream Parlour in Oak Park, Illinois, a tradition dating back to 1919.

- The **University of Wisconsin** in Madison produces 20,000 lbs per day of dairy products for campus restaurants and dormitories, including unusual ice creams like Buttermint Toffee, Orange Custard Chocolate Chip, and Cherry Chocolate Cake.

- Beginning as a dairy in Leeds, Alabama, in 1922, Spruiell Dairy has been making its **Vanilla Fudge** ice cream for three generations.

- Arthur's of Dallas sprinkles in chocolate chips to simulate seeds in its **watermelon ice.**

- The Red Fox Tavern, a country inn located in Middleburg, Virginia, since 1728, serves a wonderful **white chocolate** ice cream.

Drinks

- Dean & DeLuca offer an oversized **chocolate bowl** that is perfect for coca, café au lait, or any number of uses for "le chocolat."

- As part of the chocolate craze, there are any number of **chocolate liqueurs** on the market, including:

  1. Chocolat Mousse Liqueur, by Duchalet
  2. Haagen-Daz Cream Liqueur, by Hiram Walker, Inc.
  3. Marie Brizard Chocolat, by Schiefflein & Co.
  4. Mozart Liqueur, "A rhapsody in chocolate," by Somerset
  5. Truffles Liqueur Du Chocolat, by Heublein
  6. Vandermint, The Original Dutch Chocolate Liqueur, by Premium

- L. L. Bean's New England cookbook details how chocolate was a Northeasterner's pantry staple a decade before the Revolutionary War. It was used by Yankees, among other ways, in making "temperance drinks," as well as a **chocolate wine**, compounded of "a pint of Sherry, or a pint and a half of Port, four ounces and a half of chocolate, six ounces of the sugar," etc.

- Chocosuisse has researched and attempted to duplicate **Xocoatl**, the original Aztec chocolate drink; here is their recipe:

  2 ½ ounces unsweetened chocolate
  3 almonds, crushed in a mortar with a pestle
  2 cups warm milk
  2 tablespoons honey
  grated rind of ½ lemon
  ¾ ounce dark rum
  ⅜ ounce arrack (coconut palm liqueur)
  dash allspice
  dash ginger

Combine chocolate, almonds, and milk and heat over a low flame until chocolate melts. Chill in refrigerator. When well chilled, place in a blender or a shaker and add honey, lemon rind, dark rum, arrack, allspice, and ginger. Beat to a froth and serve.

- Billed as the **"Yuppie Drink of the 1980s,"** chocolate sodas were actually introduced by the Canfield Company of Chicago in 1971. Canfield's Diet Chocolate Fudge soda entered the fitness era with competition, though, like Famous Amos Diet Chocolate Soda, Corr's Natural White Chocolate Soda, Diet Chocolate Sundae Soda, Diet Rocky Road Soda, Diet Shasta Chocolate Fudge Soda, Vess Diet Chocolate Fudge Soda, Vintage Diet Chocolate Fudge soda, and Yoo Hoo Diet Chocolate Fudge Soda.

CHOCOLATE CLUBS

- **Chocolate clubs** became fashionable in London in the mid-seventeenth century, where social and literary figures met to gossip and drink "jocalette," as Samuel Pepys called it. In 1660, the British Parliament passed a law so every gallon of chocolate made and sold would have a duty attached to it. Hence, early chocolate consumption was enjoyed almost exclusively by the elite.

- Many of the original **chocolate houses** of the seventeenth century later became famous as clubs–like White's Chocolate House, adjoining St. James's Palace in London, or the "Cocoa Tree" Club, 64 St. James Street, Piccadilly.

- You can secure membership in the **Chocolate Lovers Association** c/o The Sweet Life in Glen Rock, New Jersey.

- *Chocolatier* offers its subscribers membership in its **Chocolate Lovers Club**, which allows discounts in the magazine's bulletin offerings. Michael Schneider is the publisher/president.

- Galerie Au Chocolat in Cincinnati offers a **chocolate-of-the-month** plan. Its children's chocolate-of-the-month service, featuring molded chocolate, has a waiting list.

- **Club Chocolat-du-Mois** in San Francisco features Belgian, French, Swiss, and American chocolatiers.

- Professional **chocolatier courses** are offered, among other places, at:

  1. New York Cooking School, 307 E. 92nd St., NY
  2. Cacoa Barry Training Center, 1500 Suckle Highway, Pennsauken, NJ
  3. Palatex, 305 E. 46th St., 5th Floor, NY

- The National Society of Chocolate Lovers, out of West Covina, California, runs **cruises to Alaska** by chocolate-flavored boat. Landry & Kling's Themes at Sea in Coral Gables, Florida (800/448-9002), also organizes annual chocolate Fantasy cruises, sponsored by the Nestle Chocolate and Confection Company. It includes a welcoming party featuring chocolates, chocolates on passengers' pillows each night, a chocolate treasure hunt, Bingo with chocolate markers and chocolate prizes, and a farewell chocolate party. A typical cruise of 200 passengers consumes about 150 cases of chocolate from 20 or more different manufacturers.

- Dr. Ray Broekel of Ipswich, Massachusetts, is founder of the **Great American Candy Bar Club**. He has an extensive collection of old and new candy bar wrappers.

- Maida Heatter, author of *The Ultimate Chocolate Book* (Knopf, 1980), bills herself as Chairperson of the Board of the Chocolate Lovers Association of the World. She says she started as a Brownie . . .

CHOCOLATE FESTIVALS

- In the May 1988 issue of *Chocolatier*, **Iris Bailin**, food editor of the *Cleveland Plain Dealer*, has a fascinating article on "What

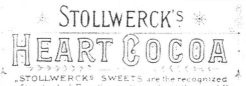

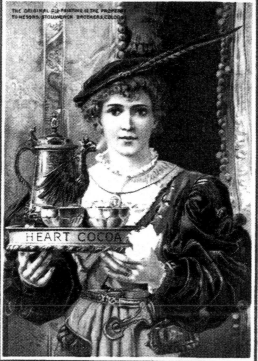

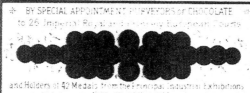

REALLY Goes on at Chocolate Festivals." She writes: "Some last a couple of hours. Others last a full day, an entire weekend, a week or longer. festivals can be pure profit-seeking ventures or charitable events. The mood can be fast-paced and packed with activities; casual, down-home and community-oriented; or elegant and sophisticated. But whatever the size, length, style or cause, the common denominator is a passion for chocolate."

- The rule for **Chocolate Expo II** at the Los Angeles Convention Center in May 1983 was said to be "survival of the fattest." More than 10,000 people paid $6.50 each; and "for the event, chocolate–the ectoplasm of their culinary fantasies–was squeezed into every conceivable, and some barely believable, forms: chocolate footprints, chocolate popcorn, chocolate ham radios, chocolate cameras, chocolate merry-go-rounds, chocolate sailboats."

–Los Angeles Times (May 15, 1983, p. 22)

- The Women's American ORT (Organization for Rehabilitation Through Training) sponsored **Chocolate Expo** in Hartford, Connecticut, in 1985 under the direction of Daniels Productions. It showcased chocolate sculptures, novelties, truffles and fudge, dietetic chocolates, and reverse chocolate cookies, with chocolate stuffed with bits of cookie.

- Disneyland Hotel Exhibition Hall in Anaheim was the scene for last year's **Chocolate Extravaganza** that benefited Children's Hospital of Orange County (CHOC). More than 10,000 chocolate lovers had a chance to participate in chocolate-eating and contests, such as "Win Your Weight in Chocolate."

- *Hershey's Great American Chocolate Festival featured a **Chocolate Fashion Show** and dessert buffet.

- **"Chocolate Funday"** was celebrated recently at the Philadelphia Zoo to benefit a new Prairie Dog Village.

- **Festivals in Taste**, a gourmet food promotion company, sponsored "The Chocolate Extraordinaire" at San Francisco's elegant

Galleria in October 1982. It featured local, national, and international chocolatiers, manufacturers, chefs, food artists, films, tastings, education, cookbooks and authors, kitchen wares, candy making, and more.

- To celebrate its annual Holiday Fare for 1985, the Fine Arts Council of Springfield, Massachusetts, sponsored **A Grand Chocolate Event** featuring a "Choco-Talk" by chocolate researcher Linda K. Fuller, continental choco-demo by cake decorator Marge Kehoe, and choco-sampling of the area's choicest restaurants and caterers.

- Chocolatetown, USA, located in Hershey, Pennsylvania, runs an annual **Great American Chocolate Festival** that is sponsored by Hershey Foods Corporation and Hotel Hershey. Meals include breakfasts of chocolate waffles, chocolate pancakes, or chocolate croissants. Later in the day you can enjoy treats like chocolate chili, chocolate chicken, chocolate salad dressing, chocolate omelets, chocolate fritters, and all sorts of gooey chocolate desserts.

- New York City's **International Chocolate Festival** of October 1983 was said to start the craze that made chocolate the food of the 1980s.

- To honor the thousand-year anniversary of its hometown of Gosselies, Belgium, Chocolaterie Bruyerre created **"Millenaire"** in 1980: a chocolate tower filled with hazelnut paste, mocha ganache, and Cointreau.

- **Mohonk Mountain House** in New Paltz, New York, held the first hotel-sponsored chocolate event in 1982, and more than a decade later its "Old-Fashioned Chocolate Weekend" continues as a favorite annual event.

- More than 20,000 people paid $7 each to attend the Los Angeles **"Salute to Chocolate"** so they could taste samples from 50 chocolatiers offering chocolate at up to $30/lb. Many of the vendors donated part of their earnings to send local handicapped athletes to the Special Olympics.

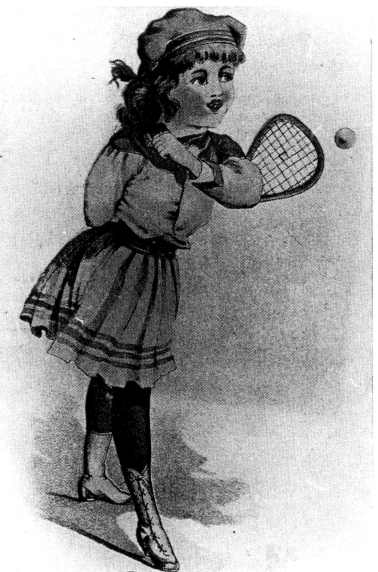

Royal Dutch Cocoa.

- Chocolate festivals are becoming a **worldwide phenomenon**. UAI Productions is planning one for Israel and many others are already scheduled far in advance. Check your chocolate media.

CHOCOLATE FUND-RAISING

- In 1660 the **British Parliament** granted a duty to Charles II on every gallon of chocolate made and sold, and during the reign of William and Mary (1690) it passed a law forbidding the sale of drinking chocolate without a license.

- The English government maintained a high import **duty** on raw cocoa beans during the seventeenth century, using chocolate as a means for increasing the country's revenue, as the Spanish had been doing for some time. The penalty for smuggling chocolate was at least one year in jail!

- **Harbor Sweets** of Marblehead, Massachusetts, has concocted specialty chocolates for several museum fund-raising events: "shawabti" (Mummy-like objects placed in the tombs of pharaohs in ancient Egypt) for the Tutankhamen exhibit at the Boston Museum of Fine Arts; a reproduction of "Old Ironsides"; ship's figurehead from the collection of Salem's Peabody Museum; miniature chocolate dinosaurs for the Carnegie Institute; Mint for the U.S. Constitution Museum; Met Solos, Met Mints, and Wunderbars for the Metropolitan Opera of New York; Orange Blossoms for the Cleveland Orchestra; chocolate milk bottles for the Boston Children's Museum; Mental Health Mints for the Massachusetts Association of Mental Health; Instru-Mints for the Lincoln Center for the Performing Arts; and many others.

- According to its publication *In celebration of seventy years . . .,* **L. S. Heath & Sons** entered the fund-raising business in 1964, selling its famous Heath Bars to clubs, schools, and other organizations for resale profits.

- **The Kosher Chocolate Factory** in Northfield, Illinois, helps schools and synagogues use its products in fund-raising events.

Besides "meichal" pops and bars, the company features "Chocolates for the Young Gourmet," boxed chocolates, and a chocolate candy-making kit.

- The cacao bean played such an important role in the religious lives of sixteenth century Aztecs, who believed the prophets had brought its seeds from Paradise, that it was considered a valuable **medium of exchange**. One hundred beans could buy a slave, four a turkey. In his *Historie of the East and West Indies*, written in 1604, Joseph Acosta writes: "The Indians used no gold nor silver to buy withall . . . and unto this day this custom continues amongst the Indians, as in the province of Mexico in steede of money they use Cocoa (which is a small fruite), and therewith buy what they will." Known as "patlache," 8,000 cacao nibs constituted one "xiquipilli."

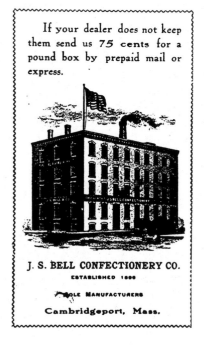
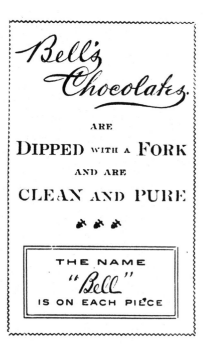

- **Munson's** Candy Kitchen in Bolton, Connecticut, uses these chocolate products as fund-raisers for groups: buttercrunch, almond bark, chocolate nonpareils, cashew caramel patties, chocolate cups, boxes and bars of chocolate, and chocolate animals.

- You can have your "organization's **name**, mascot's name, or candidate's name" molded onto Harry London's (North Canton, Ohio) quality chocolate bar for personalized fund-raising programs.

- The **Peekskill (New York) Area Health Center** baked a world-record chocolate chip cookie as its fund-raiser. Using 1.2 million chocolate chips, 340 pounds of flour, 250 pounds of sugar, 200 pounds of shortening, and 750 eggs that were all donated by Entenmann's Bakery of Bay Shore, Long Island, the cookie was made to serve 6,000 people–at $1 each.

- Cocoa beans were originally used as an exchange commodity during times of **slavery**: "If the need to buy a human body was for a more transitory purpose, the price was better. The services of certain Mayan women could be had for a mere eight to ten cacao beans a night" (Kolpas, 1978, p. 16).

- UAI Productions presented "A Salute to Chocolate II" at the Los Angeles Convention Center in May 1984 to help the **TriValley Special Olympics**. Fund-raising activities included a celebrity auction of chocolate creations, a drawing for a gift certificate to a chocolate cruise, raffles, guessing your weight in chocolate, and special discounts on chocolates and ice cream.

- The "King of Chocolate Fund-Raising," **World's Finest Chocolate, Inc**. of Chicago was founded in 1940 by Edmond Opler, Sr. The company maintains a large professional staff that helps groups involved in charitable events and promotions. With a newly renovated chocolate manufacturing plant, World's Finest can produce a million chocolate bars for fund-raising every day.

CHOCOLATE MARKETING

- Chocolate **boutiques** are springing up everywhere, as accessible as ice cream parlours, and fashionable stores like Saks Fifth

Avenue, Bloomingdales, and Macy's are carrying full lines of gourmet chocolates.

- Robert B. Finn, Vice President and General Manager of the Bulk Chocolate and Franchise Divisions for Nestle Company, reported in 1983 that **boxed chocolates** were being purchased 50% more often than they had been six years previously. These purchases fall mostly in the gift sector, "reflecting successful promotion by industry members," and are being bought more regularly for in-home consumption.

  –The Boxed Chocolates Market 1983: A Report on Consumer Behavior, Nestle

- Sandra Boynton reports that her **breakthrough greeting card** for Recycled Paper Products was her 1976 design of a sensuous, forlorn hippo bemoaning, "Things are getting worse–send chocolate."

- In 1824, **John Cadbury** opened a coffee and tea business in Birmingham, England, and he carried cocoa beans as a sideline. As part of his merchandising, he offered window displays of his cocoa bean grindings.

- **Cailler Chocolate** markets itself as "The Preferred Chocolate of Switzerland."

- An even stronger motto comes from **Charbonnel et Walker** of England: "Probably the best chocolates in the world."

- According to the U.S. Department of Commerce, the greatest gains in the candy industry have been realized recently in the **chocolate category**, especially the assorted/boxed kind and especially imports. Channels of distribution tend to be shifting away from drug stores to specialty and department stores.

- The **chocolate-flavor** business in the United States is a $25 million industry.

- The first scholarly academic report on the chocolate phenomenon, **"Choco-Marketing-Mania,"** was presented by Dr. Linda

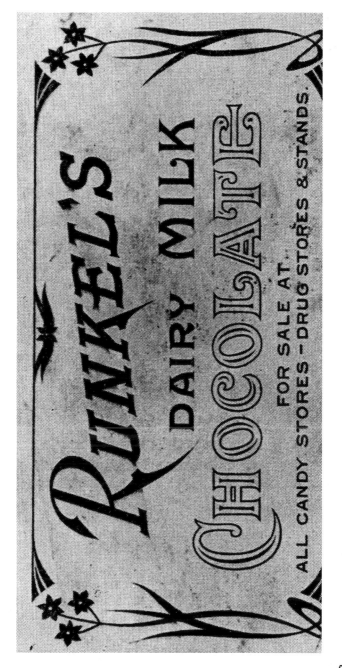

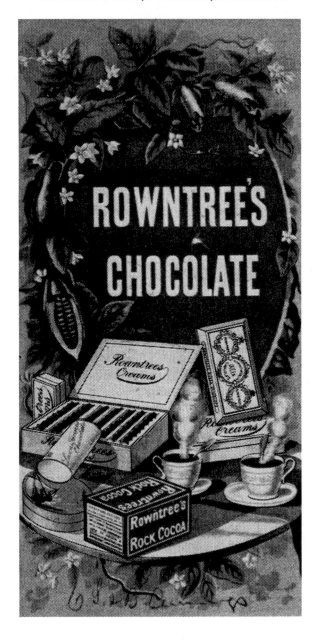

K. Fuller to the Popular Culture Association in Louisville, Kentucky, in April 1985.

- Winters Chocolatier uses a 24-hour telephone service called the **"Chocolate Menu,"** whereby customers can place their orders by numbers and names of various chocolates.

- Sweden's **Cloetta** chocolate "designer bars" are packaged in denim-decorator wrappers.

- Documenting the extraordinary increase in **cocoa consumption** at the turn of the century, Walter Baker and Company credited the following:
  1. A reduction in the retail price, bringing it within the means of the poorer classes;
  2. A more general recognition of the value of cocoa as an article of food; and
  3. Improvements in methods of preparation by which it is adapted to the wants of different classes of consumers.

  –Cocoa and Chocolate, 1910.

- For its faithful customers like Cartier, Rolex, Rolls Royce, Mercedes Benz, and Piaget, Moreau Chocolates of Switzerland creates specially shaped chocolates such as watches or cars that can be given as **corporate gifts**.

- **Double Truffle Chocolates** bills itself as a contribution to world peace. The Beverly Hills company claims its truffles "have been used to ease family tensions and office squabbles, but recently they've been called upon to make an even greater contribution. Certain advisors to world leaders have been suggesting that they might even be used to soothe international tensions . . . possibly even avert wars."

- With liquor sales in restaurants slipping, many places are pushing **fancy chocolate desserts** priced at 300-400+% above cost. For example, Pillsbury's Bennigan Chain recently introduced "Death by Chocolate," and Franco's Hidden Harbor in Seattle just added ten chocolate desserts such as "Chocolate Decadence Cake" for $4.50.

- **Godiva Chocolatier** is responsible for breaking the $3/lb barrier in chocolate sales. The company took the tack of introducing their chocolates as the most elegant and most expensive chocolates available–and it worked!

- *The Indian Nectar, or a Discourse Concerning Chocolate*, a book written during the reign of Charles II of England, suggested that the best chocolate could be purchased from a man named Mortimer of East Smithfield "for 6s. 8d. per pound, and commoner sorts for about half that price."

- The Chocolate Manufacturers Association of the U.S.A. claims that "chocolate and confectionery industries provide about 60,000 production **jobs** and an estimated 240,000 additional jobs supporting the production and sales of chocolate and confectionery foods."

  –"Chocolate: Nutritional and Economic Short Takes"

- The Associated Press reported (August 7, 1984) on a **Korean delicatessen** owner on Park Avenue in New York City who wanted to placate his unwelcoming neighbors. He decided to display imported chocolates in the middle of the store when he learned that the key opposition leader liked them.

- From 1980-83, the period when high-priced, upscale **luxury chocolate** began, there was a 16% increase in chocolate in the United States–to 2.18 billion pounds. The latest figures from the U.S. Department of Commerce show a 21% increase since 1980, to $9 billion in chocolate sales.

- **Mail-order chocolate** combines two incredible phenomena of the 1980s. Nearly every major chocolate manufacturer has cashed in on the convenience, personalized service, and specialized offerings that mail order can offer. Most, however, will only ship chocolate in weather-appropriate seasons.

- The person singled out as most responsible for the current interest in chocolate in the United States is **Al Pechenik**, who, when hired as president of Godiva Chocolates when it was bought by Campbell Soups Company in 1966, decided to upgrade chocolate–raising the price to $20/lb and advertising it as an expensive, special treat. Godiva staffed its chocolate boutiques with uniformed attendants who talked to customers about their "chocolate needs," and who packaged their purchases in deluxe gold-roped boxes. Pechenik later headed up Michel Guerard, and now is reportedly working for Poulain.

- "Chocolate was, in those days (nineteenth century), primarily a beverage, and to it were attributed many **qualities**; indeed, it was considered an aphrodisiac, a digestive, a soporific, a tonic, even a cure for certain intestinal afflictions."

  –Susan Heller Anderson, "Making Chocolates in the Artisan's Way," *New York Times* (December 17, 1980)

- Citing its nutrient value, Runkel's Cocoa, established in 1870, announced: "**Pale People Take Notice:** from the above facts you will understand why persons who are pale, 'run down,' or recovering from illness, are greatly benefited by Runkel's Cocoa. To help regain their strength, they should drink one cupful of Runkel's every day at eleven and one at four o'clock as well as with their meals."

- According to Lesly Berger, author of *The Gourmet's Guide to Chocolate* (Quill, 1984), "We are in the midst of a **chocolate renaissance**, a veritable confectionery age of enlightenment" in terms of all the chocolate products that are available.

- The first chocolate sold in the **retail market** was in 1657 when a Frenchman opened a shop in London where solid chocolate for making a "frothy chocolate beverage" could be purchased for 10-15 shillings.

- **S.E. Rykoff & Co.** of Los Angeles, "Foods and Cookware of Distinction since 1911," has a clever advertisement that reads: "Our Chocolate is to Die for. Any Volunteers?"

- "Selling Krön chocolates at up to $30 a pound is not just selling candy; it's **selling an umlaut!**"

  –Jerry Adler et al., "America's Chocolate Binge,"
  Newsweek (April 4, 1983), pp. 50+

- Some familiar chocolate bar **slogans:**

  1. "It's the great American, great American chocolate bar." (Hershey Bar)
  2. "Sometimes you feel like a nut; sometimes you don't." (Almond Joy and Mounds)
  3. "N-E-S-T-L-E-S, Nestle makes the very best . . . chocolate." (Nestle Crunch)
  4. "Two great tastes in one candy bar." (Reese's Peanut Butter Cups)

- Brown and Haley, makers of Almond Roca, used to insert **"Smart Cards,"** containing jokes, trivia, puzzles, and cartoons, in their chocolate Mountain Bars.

- Happily, chocolate **sources** are emerging everywhere: fairs and festivals, department stores, gourmet food shops, airports, chocolate boutiques, and numerous mail-order outlets.

- In 1979, Americans **spent** $14 million on chocolates; in 1982, more than $50 million; last year that figure was $9 billion.

- "People can be taught to pay $25 or more a pound for a product they had always bought in 25-cent portions at the drugstore. **Status-wary shoppers** found that if chocolate cost enough, it was okay to give it as a gift."

  –Sam Maddox, "U.S. coming out of the chocolate closet," *Advertising Age* (September 27, 1984)

- The oldest grocery **trademark** in the United States is claimed by Baker's Chocolate: "The Beautiful Chocolate Girl," a painting which hangs today in the Dresdan Art Gallery. "Trademarks have a certain value in themselves," says Raimo Hertto, Executive Vice President of Finland's Huhtamaki, which bought Good

& Plenty, Clark Bars, and Milk Duds in 1983 (*Wall Street Journal*, June 13, 1985). A number of companies join them in resurrecting old favorites, like Nestle's purchase and upgrading of Oh Henry!, Goobers, Raisinets, and Chunky.

- **Trade organizations** serving the chocolate industry can be found in England, Mexico, France, Switzerland, and the United States.

- "My **view of the market** is quite simply: Are our cookies incredibly fabulous? Yes. Do they make people happy? Yes. Are they as good as homemade? In my opinion, yes. Do people love to eat them? Yes. Are they going to give up the things they love to eat? I think that's very doubtful . . . I mean, really, if something is fresh, warm, and wonderful and it makes you feel good, are you going to stop buying cookies? You grew up with cookies. Your mom made you cookies."

> –Debbi Fields/Mrs. Fields Chocolate Chippery, Inc.
> (July 1984)

- Finding out that 18- to 34-year olds eat candy more than 20 times a year, marketers are zeroing in on **young adults** in their advertising campaigns. The television commercial for Nestle's Crunch, for example, features basketball player Kareem Abdul-Jabbar, while its Alpine bar is being run in magazines like *Cosmopolitan* and *GQ*. Hershey is advertising its Skor bar in the *New Yorker* and other upscale magazines as the kind of chocolate bar that King Henry VIII would enjoy.

CHOCOLATE MEDIA

- From 1979-1992 these **American publications** have run feature articles about chocolate: *Ad Forum, Advertising Age, Adweek's Marketing Week, Americana, American Legion, Americas, Back Stage, Barrons, Bazaar, Better Homes and Gardens, Beverage Industry, Bicycling, Black Enterprise, Boston Magazine, Business Week, Canadian Consumer, Candy Industry, Chain Store*

Age Executive, Changing Times, Chemical & Engineering News, Chicago, Childhood Education, Chocolatier, Christian Science Monitor, Colorado Business Magazine, Consumer Reports, Cosmopolitan, Crain's Chicago Business, Crain's New York Business, Cuisine, Current Health, Direct Marketing, Discover, Dynamic Years, Ebony, The Economist, FDA Consumer, Financial World, Food Development, Food Processing, Food Product Development, Food Technology, Fortune, Gifts & Decorative Accessories, Good Housekeeping, Gourmet, Harpers Bazaar, Health, History Today, Horticulture, House and Garden, House Beautiful, Independent Restaurants, Instructor, Journal of Commerce and Commercial, Library Journal, Life, Los Angeles, Mademoiselle, Madison Avenue, Management Today, Marketing and Media Decisions, Minneapolis-St. Paul, Money, Moneysworth, Mother Earth News, National Geographic, Nation's Business, Nation's Restaurant News, New England Business, New Scientist, New Statesman and Society, Newsweek, New York, New York Times, New York Times Book Review, Packaging Digest, People Weekly, Philadelphia, Popular Photographer, Prevention, Progressive Grocer, Publishers Weekly, Reader's Digest, Redbook, Restaurant Business Magazine, Restaurant Hospitality, Restaurants and Institutions, Sales and Marketing Management, San Francisco, San Francisco Business Times, Savvy, School Library Journal, Science News, Seventeen, Smithsonian, Southern Living, Sport, Sunset, Supermarket, Texas Monthly, Time, Town and Country, Trailer Boats, Travel-Holiday, U.S.A. Today, U.S. Distribution Journal, U.S. News & World Report, U.S. Tobacco and Candy Journal, Vogue, Wall Street Journal, Washingtonia, Washington Post, Weight Watchers, Wilson Library Bulletin, and Working Woman.

- Early in the 1980s, nearly every major **book publishing firm** released at least seven cookbooks, and had a full complement of chocolate cookbooks ready for release after the successes of Sandra Boynton's *Chocolate, the Consuming Passion* (600,000 copies sold) and Maida Heatter's *Book of Great Chocolate Desserts* (175,000 sold).

- *The Boston Gazette and Country Journal* carried the first notice of the sale of cocoa and chocolate in the United States on March 12, 1770:

  To be sold by
  JOHN BAKER
  At his store in Back Street a few Bags of
  the best cocoa; also choice Chocolate by
  the Hundred or Smaller Quantity.

- On January 16, 1985, journalist Bob Greene of the *Chicago Tribune* wrote a blurb about a tasty diet chocolate soda he'd tried; within days a national craze developed for **Canfield's Diet Chocolate Fudge Soda**. The product is totally artificial: it contains two calories per can, no sodium, no caffeine–and no chocolate. Yet, people began to send the 62-year-old Canfield Beverage Company of Chicago blank checks for cases of the stuff, while others called in from Canada to China, and reportedly a Canfield truck driver was pulled over by a state patrolman who wanted to know how he could get the soda for his wife. Within a week, more than a million cans, the total of what had been sold the previous year, were sold out from local distributorships; within four months, 51 million cans had been sold, and 46 licensing agreements had been signed. What a powerful combination: chocolate and the media.

- It has been noted that when a magazine has **chocolate on the cover**, sales typically double.

- Adrienne Trouw of Holland Handicrafts in Davis, California, has a collection of 350 antique **chocolate molds** that have been featured in several magazine articles.

- *Chocolate News* called itself the "World's Favorite Flavor Publication." Established in 1981 by Milton Zelman, the New York newsletter was printed on chocolate-colored pages and was mailed to 8,500 subscribers. Its mission was "to heighten chocolate consciousness . . . to expedite the chocolate cravings of our readers."

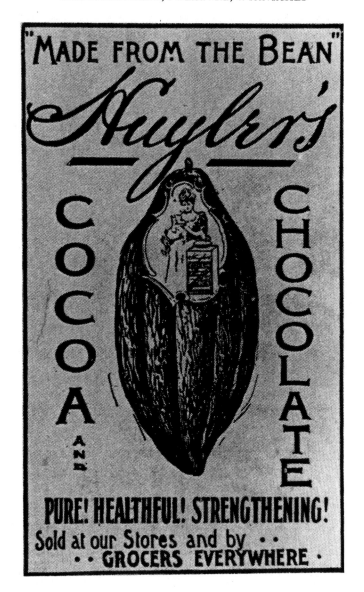

- "The magazine for gourmet chocolate lovers," *Chocolatier* made its appearance under the Haymarket Group, Ltd. of New York in 1983; already it has 125,000 subscribers in 30 countries. While it began as a quarterly, interest has been such that it has been a bimonthly magazine since 1986. Information on both current subscriptions and back issues are available c/o the editor at 45 West 34th Street, New York.

- Marlene Tanzer ran a weekly syndicated newspaper column devoted strictly to **"Choc Talk."**

- Chocolate first appeared in the **cinema** when Jean Harlow ate some candy in the 1933 comedy *Dinner at Eight*. In 1936, Alfred Hitchcock's *The Secret Agent* included a spy chase through a Swiss chocolate factory with John Gielgud and Peter Lorre. Bette Davis used chocolate in her 1950 *All About Eve* to provide self-gratification, while Gregory Peck used it to hide a secret message for Sophia Loren in *Arabesque*. In the 1976 mystery *Marathon Man*, Roy Scheider as the double agent hid secret material between layers of Godiva chocolates, while in the same year James Coco as a sleuth in Neil Simon's *Murder By Death* reprimanded his chauffeur for getting him chocolate with raisins rather than nuts. Chocolate was the star of the 1978 film *Who Is Killing the Great Chefs of Europe?*, where Jacqueline Bisset laced her Bombe Richelieu with double-deep chocolate and raspberry liqueur.

- A timely Ziegler cartoon in the *New Yorker* (10/14/91) shows three couples munching desserts while one notes, "Who could have imagined that such a wonderful recipe for brownies would be hidden away in the **Dead Sea Scrolls**?"

- In a study of "The Chocolate and Gourmet Food Markets," J. K. Fuchs and Associates (New Rochelle, New York, 1983) found the following **epicurean magazines** placing an increasing emphasis on chocolate: *Bon Appetit, Cuisine, Food and Wine, Gourmet,* and *The Cook's Magazine.*

- The first public notice of the manufacture of chocolate in the United States appeared June 18, 1771, in the Massachusetts' *Essex Gazette:*

  AMOS TRASK,
  At his House a little below the Bell-Tavern in
  DANVERS,
  Makes and sells CHOCOLATE,
  Which he will warrant to be good, and takes
  Cocoa to grind. Those who may please to
  favor him with their custom may depend
  upon being well served, and at a very cheap
  Rate.

- *How Do They Make Chocolate,* a four-minute film produced in 1970, stars Woody Allen and Jo Anne Worley. Produced by NBC-TV for children, it is available for sale or rent from Films Incorporated of Wilmette, Illinois.

- Comic-strip characters Archie, Reggie, Veronica, and Jughead's favorite hangout is **"Pop's Choklit Shoppe."**

- More than a century after it had been used in Spain, the first announcement of cocoa's introduction into England appeared on June 16, 1657, in the *Public Advertiser:* "In Bishopsgate Street, in Queen's Head Alley, at a Frenchman's house, is an excellent West Indian drink, called chocolate, to be sold, where you may have it ready at any time; and also unmade, at reasonable rates."

- Dudley-Anderson-Yutzy of New York is the **public relations** agency for the Chocolate Manufacturers of America, which is located in McLean, Virginia.

- Former *Chocolatier* editor **Joan Steuer** is described as eating chocolate by the pound: "a $600 Monopoly set, computers, tennis balls, dog biscuits, a Noah's ark, a 5,000-calorie pig, a picture of herself, fettucini, pizza, croissants, and Merv Griffin's ear."

Actually, she's a slim, blonde, 26-year-old dedicated choco-journalist whose ideal dessert is "outrageously deep and dark."
–Peggy Brawley, "Magazine Editor Joan Steuer's Consuming Passion is Chocolate," *People* (May 21, 1984), pp. 105-6.

- For the 100th performance of *Sugar Babies* on Broadway, Mickey Rooney and Ann Miller were presented with solid chocolate life-sized busts of themselves, sculpted by James Victor of A. Panache of Philadelphia.

- *Willie Wonka and the Chocolate Factory* is considered the classic chocolate-lovers' movie. This 1971 film, starring the zany Gene Wilder, offered a lifetime of chocolate and a tour of Willie Wonka's "Kingdom of Taste" to the lucky finders of five golden tickets inside Wonka Bars. A particular feature of the film was the introduction of the "Gobstopper," a never-ending hard candy.

CHOCOLATE NOVELTIES

- Harbor Sweets of Marblehead, MA, has devised an **advent calendar** that has a chocolate treat behind each of the doors in anticipation of December 25.

- Charles of the Ritz has developed a $20 **Aroma Disc Player** that can give you the sweet smells of "Chocolate After Dinner Mints"–a good no-cal alternative for a chocolate fix!

- Seattle artist/sculptor Gus Gosanko has developed a **Chocolate Art** business, using custom molds to create lifelike animals (lions, tigers, bears, gorillas, seafaring life, and even a Tyrannosaurus Rex) and other unusual configurations.

- If the recession and car payments are getting you down, try treating yourself to any number of chocolate **automobiles** that are available at the confectionery of your choice.

- It looks like a bottle of **Bordeux wine**, but Bissinger's of St. Louis has produced a bottle stuffed with European milk chocolate creams, foil-wrapped to resemble corks.

- With a single chocolate theme, the **Boulder Calendar Company** in Colorado puts out "Schokolade," a calendar depicting gourmet chocolate.

- Executive Sweet of Bellaire, Texas, features chocolate chip cookies that come packaged in boxes designed to look like **briefcases**.

- Chocolateers of San Francisco produces a **bumper sticker** warning: "I brake for chocolates."

- **Chocolate Byte** is available from The Chocolate Software Company of Los Angeles–a 5 1/4", 4.8 ounce "floppy disk" of milk chocolate. Want a byte?

- Smile, you're on **Candied Camera!** Toha Trading, Inc. of Los Angeles makes chocolate cameras, chocolate calculators, chocolate typewriters, chocolate cassette players, and chocolate computers.

- **Candles** resembling chocolate ice cream sundaes can be ordered from Epistrof, Inc. of New York.

- Harry London's Gourmet Chocolate of North Canton, Ohio, puts out **Candy Store Aprons** imprinted with 24 reasons to eat chocolate.

- The Great Northwestern Greeting Seed Company (800/992-GROW), which prints its **cards** on recycled paper, offers packets of chocolate mix with them for making creamy milkshakes or rich, hot chocolate.

- *The Chef's Catalog* from Northbrook, Illinois, "Professional Restaurant Equipment for the Home Chef," specializes in chocolate-related supplies: computer recipe discs, books, videos, molds, spatula, thermometer, truffle scoop, sauces, and a "Do-it Yourself" kit.

- **"Choc-O-Bar,"** a 1-3/4-oz vitamin-enriched taste treat for dogs, is manufactured by Redi, available for 98 cents at pet supply stores.

- Essentially Chocolates of Washington, D.C., puts out the **Choco-holic Gift Basket**–$39.50 for a collection of milk and dark chocolates, cocoa, Baci, truffles, and lots more.

- **Choco-holic Relief Spray**™ is a 7-oz aerosol spray available from Choco-holics Unanimous.

- Krön Chocolatier of New York not only IS one, but has created a **chocolate angel** for you–a $60, 5-3/4 pounder in milk, dark, or white chocolate.

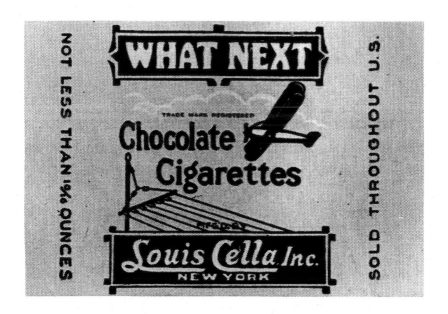

- For $10,000, you can have Lenotre of Paris sculpt a two-foot solid **chocolate bust** of you. You merely supply them with photographs of yourself from several angles–and the check.

- You can get a **chocolate calling card**, a 5″ × 7″ chocolate block with your name and credentials on it, from Kilwin's Candy Kitchen in Petoskey, Michigan.

- Butterfly in New York offers a "split" of St. Moritz **chocolate champagne**–12 ounces of solid milk chocolate, guaranteed hangover-proof.

- Astor Chocolate Company of Glendale, New York, puts out a "Winner Eats All" solid **chocolate chess set**, made of 3 lbs of white and dark chocolate, for $70. Or maybe you'd prefer to play **chocolate dominoes**, with dark and white chocolate pieces. Karl Bissinger (800/325-8881) also offers a 30-piece regulation set of white chocolate dominoes.

- The Kitchen Crate of New York offers a **Chocolate Chipper Set** that is billed as being able to "turn a ton of chocolate into a tower of chips in minutes." The chipper has metal prongs and a hardware handle, and comes with a 10″ square maple board.

- Rudi's of Woburn, Massachusetts, has a $25 **"Chocolate Chocolate Box,"** loaded with fudgy truffles, mint-flavored cocoa, praline chocolate seashells, chocolate-covered pistachios, and more.

- Penyak's Patties in Statesville, North Carolina, has **chocolate Christmas ornaments** and greeting cards.

- Remember those **chocolate cigarettes** you used to pretend to puff on as a kid? Now you can buy Pushpinoff's Coco Golds, packed in a snazzy case.

- **Chocolate Collection** in St. Paul produces T-shirts announcing "I can be had–try chocolate" and "Give me chocolate or give me death," a mug proclaiming "Viva La Chocolat!", and an apron with 50 answers to the question, "Chocolate, How Do I Love Thee?"

- M.Y.T. Trading Company of Carson, California, puts out a **chocolate comb**–the ideal way to get snarls out.

- **Chocolate Decadence Sauce**–chocolate raspberry decadence, chocolate orange decadence, or chocolate caramel decadence come in 16-oz jars from Narsai's Market in Kensington, California.

- The James Beard Collection, a not-for-profit organization in Darnestown, Maryland, includes "chocolate" ice cream cone **earrings** and a cake server page marker.

- The Sweet Life, Inc. of Glen Rock, New Jersey, puts out an annual **Chocolate Engagement Calendar** that features chocolate data and designs.

- **Chocolate Lace** in Danbury, Connecticut, produces its intricate chocolate lace in dark, chocolate mint, or toasted almond milk chocolate flavors.

- Inviting customers to tempt their lovers with the ultimate in sweet talk is Melvin Schechter, founder of **The Chocolate Letter** in New York City. For about $20, his company will mold and mail up to 90 words on a 5″ × 8″ half-pound slab of dark or milk chocolate. While most of his greetings have centered around seasonal/love holidays, there have been orders for a poison-pen letter, religious messages, congratulations for giving up smoking, letters of job resignations, etc.

- To prevent refrigerator raids, put up some mock **chocolate magnets**, available from Cricket Designs in San Jose, California.

- Bissinger's of Cincinnati offers a **chocolate mill** that is perfect for decorating cakes, cookies, frostings, and parfaits.

- A **chocolate mink coat** can be ordered from Long Grove (Illinois) Confectionery; it's 14 oz of milk chocolate, trimmed in dark chocolate.

- Love Chocolate Factory in Hartsville, Ohio, specializes in **chocolate molds**.

- A sweet, stuffed **Chocolate Moose** toy is available from Dakin of San Francisco.

- As part of a special request for someone who had a nose job, Dreams Come True of Pittsburgh has invented a **chocolate nose.**

- Sweets, Inc. puts out a **chocolate pacifier** for any chocolate baby.

- Pasta machines for making **chocolate pasta** are available at Macy's in New York, The Emporium in San Francisco, and Gimbels in the Midwest.

- Double Truffle Chocolates of Beverly Hills have had great success with their **chocolate pâté.** The dark chocolate, with a taste of Grand Marnier, comes in a silver-plated reusable oyster shell.

- **Chocolate Photos** emboss your face in milk or dark chocolate, made by child psychiatrist and chocolate entrepreneur Dr. Victor Syrmis of New York. Send him a black-and-white or color photo, which he will turn into a foil mold. He's already done Nancy Reagan, Henny Youngman, Calvin Klein, Joan Rivers, and Lena Hornel, among others. A box of 24 pieces, each wrapped in gold foil, costs about $35. Chocolate Photos' slogan is "We put your face in chocolate from a photograph." The company has received "every conceivable photograph," according to Syrmis, "from ordinary people to pets, trees, plants, transvestites, and nudity." He tells of a woman who ordered hundreds of chocolate photos of herself and her husband, then melted them in honor of their divorce.

- Sin Bad Sweets of Clovis, California, produces a phenomenal **chocolate phyllo.**

- Cailler puts out the ideal host/hostess snack: **Choco Pic**, a combination of Swiss fruit and nuts coated with chocolate.

- To satisfy any number of crazy cravings, Figi's of Marshfield, Wisconsin, offers **chocolate pickles**–a 9-1/2-oz jar of green-foiled milk chocolate oblongs. At Eastertime, Figi's features an "Egg Crate" of chocolate eggs.

- Not only are **chocolate pill dispensers** available from Chocolate By Design, you can actually fill them with chocolate aspirins!

- At Munson's Candy Kitchen in Bolton, Connecticut, you can get a **chocolate pizza**: it has a chocolate base, topped with cherries and walnuts, then drizzled all over with white chocolate.

- **Chocolate popcorn** makes a delightful movie-viewing snack; it's available at The Popcorn Factory in Lake Bluff, Illinois.

- Celestial Arts in Berkeley, California, offers by mail order a "Give Me Chocolate or Give Me Death" **chocolate poster** that features a chocoholic's quiz, chocolate calorie chart, and other humorous items. Chocolate posters dating from the turn of the century through the 1950s are also available from New York art dealer Phyllis Elliot.

- Joan Shevell of New Rochelle, NY, offers a unique dessert idea: the "Mousseketeer," a **chocolate punchbowl**, atop a chocolate platter, filled with chocolate mousse, surrounded by chocolate cups–so when the mousse is gone, cleanup is easy.

- It may be the same by any name, but a **chocolate rose** from Another Estie in Northridge, California, can be made out of white, milk, or dark chocolate. Edible chocolate roses are also available from Rowe-Manse Emporium of Clifton, NJ, Chocolate Fantasies of Clovis, CA, and many other places. **Chocolate chip roses** are available through Unforgettable of Los Angeles.

- You can get a 17″ **chocolate Santa Claus** filled with five pounds of jelly beans at Mother Myrick's Ice Cream Parlor and Fudge Factory in Manchester, Vermont.

- As part of its Chocolate-of-the-Month plan, Galerie au Chocolat of Cincinnati sends its January customers some **chocolate sardines**, solid milk chocolate wrapped in foil and sealed in a real tin.

- Orange Tree Imports of Madison, Wisconsin, features **chocolate scratch-and-sniff stickers** in its chocolate collection.

- Colossus Corporation of New Haven, Connecticut, manufactures **chocolate soap cookies**–chocolate chip and pseudo-chip.

- Jheri Redding Products, a division of Conair Corporation, puts out a **chocolate styling gel** with "beautiful hold and control for brunettes."

- Gilles 1840 produces both **chocolate tea and chocolate coffee**.

- "The Met by Mail," located on New York City's Broadway, offered **chocolate tickets** for "Opening Night at the Met."

- Orvis, "A Sporting Tradition since 1856," has a mail-order catalogue out of Manchester, Vermont, that is geared to the outdoorsman/gourmand; it offers a **chocolate trout**.

- Triple M Productions of Fair Oaks, California, has produced **"Chocolates by Video,"** with step-by-step demonstrations for creating turtles, English toffee, truffles, etc. for VHS/BETAs.

- Byteware, Inc. makes chocolate **"Circuit Chips,"** 7-oz replicas of computer chips that are labeled as "the chocolate computer buffs love to byte."

- McStevens of Clackamus, Oregon, makes **cocoa** in several unusual flavors, including: cherry, orange, spice, mint, amaretto, and Kahlua.

- Gabrielle's Fine Chocolates of Maywood, New Jersey, has some unusual **edible containers** for its Belgian-style chocolates: a chocolate clam shell, 7" round chocolate box, chocolate Yule Log, chocolate Dutch shoe, and chocolate heart-shaped boxes.

- Catherine's Chocolates of Great Barrington, Massachusetts, puts out **"corporate head"**–a pure milk chocolate bust of an executive, complete with pin-striped suit and tie. It's the ideal way to chew off someone else's head!

- Zoria Farms of San Jose ships chocolate-covered **dried fruit** from September through April; choose from apricots, prunes, peaches, pears, or a mixed fruit combination.

- Although drinking chocolate was a well-established activity by the latter part of the nineteenth century, **"eating chocolate,"** introduced by Fry and Sons of England in 1847, was still somewhat of a novelty in its day.

- **"Edible Compliments"** are chocolate molds manufactured by Jareen Company of Los Angeles. They come in a number of fun shapes: fish, baby corn, hearts, bunnies, flowers, even a breadbasket.

- ADI of Glendale, New York, has produced miniature **erasers** to simulate chocolate bars like Mr. Goodbar, Krackel, Hershey's, Reese's, etc.

- **"Escargots,"** chocolate snail shells molded in milk chocolate and striped with dark chocolate, then filled with praline paste, are available through Stork's Pastry Shop in Whitestone, New York.

- The Peninsula Hotel in Hong Kong offers this unique guest service: imported swiss chocolates–Cointreau and Kirsch-filled–are available by **FAX**, elegantly packaged in a bellhop's hatbox.

- Sweet Assets of Grosse Pointe, Michigan, produces a product called **"Financial Crunch,"**–eleven (a "banker's dozen") silver dollar-shaped milk chocolate crispies.

- **Fondue au Chocolat** is available from Splendid Chocolates in gourmet and specialty shops–$8 for a 10-1/2-oz package of Belgian milk or dark chocolate ready to be melted for your favorite fruit, biscuits, cake, whatever. Chocolate **fondue forks** are sold by Bridge Kitchenware Corporation in New York City.

- Knights, Ltd. offers a **French bistro clock** that reads "CHOCO-LAT de la BELLE FRANCE."

- Enter a contest with your own chocolate-scented **Frisbee**, produced by SuedeCraft Enterprises, Inc. of Willowbrook, Illinois.

- **"Chocolate Fudge"** can be obtained as a perfume for the ladies or a 1/2-oz bottle of cologne for men from Nikke Distributing of Minneapolis. (Note: I've ordered it–it does smell like chocolate!)

- The Silver Palate of New York, which has two best-selling cookbooks on the market, also offers its fantastic **fudge sauces** for sale–flavors such as caramel fudge, raspberry fudge, Grand Marnier fudge, and hazelnut fudge.

- You can get a chocolate **garbage can** at Rohr in Geneva; you can fill it with some of their other products: chocolate tennis balls, chocolate champagne bottles filled with truffles or griottes, Petite Marmite chocolate kettles, chocolate spools of thread, and much more.

- **Godiva** puts out a number of novelty chocolates, like chocolate golf balls, chocolate shotgun shells, a chocolate tennis ball tin, and many other exciting items.

- Long Grove (Illinois) Confectionery produces a 15-lb chocolate **gorilla**.

- Chocolate **greeting cards**, with or without messages, are available from Recycled Products, Godiva, Krön, and many other companies. Sweetvisions Publishing Company in Newton Highlands, Massachusetts, issues "Sweetness and Light" chocolate notecards, while Swiss Colony offers personalized Currier and Ives milk chocolate greeting cards. California Dreamers of Chicago produces amusing ones with such messages as "Nobody knows the truffles I've seen" and "With liberty and chocolate for all."

- Nautical motifs are just one specialty offered by **Harbor Sweets** of Marblehead, Massachusetts. Try their Sweet Sloop sailboat, caramel-filled Sand Dollar, boat-embossed peppermint Marblehead Mint, or chocolate Barque Sarah, named for local ships from the 1850s. Harbor Sweets was the official chocolatier of the 1984 America's Cup yacht races.

- The Neiman-Marcus Epicure Shop in Boston sells a hollow chocolate life-sized human-shaped **head** for about $100.

- Hershey Foods Corporation has put out a whole line of **Hershey's Chocolate Memories**, a collection of tins decorated with oldtime advertisements and recipes.

- Ebullience Perfume Company of Philadelphia has developed a product called **"Hot Chocolate"** cologne for men; it comes packaged in a cocoa tin.

- Ideal Toys produces **Kisses**, a teddy bear with a T-shirt sporting a Hershey Bar logo and guaranteed to maintain a chocolate aroma for two years.

- Pazzaz, Inc. of Los Angeles puts out chocolate-oriented **kitchen magnets** such as Nestle's Crunch, Tootsie Rolls, Milk Duds, Oreos, etc.

- **Koko Kong** is a six-pound solid Belgian milk chocolate "sweet gorilla" that comes caged in a crate, deliverable from Helen Grace Chocolates of Lynwood, California.

- Chap Stick produces a "Chewy Chocolate" **lip stick**; Minnetonka, Inc. has Chocolate Creams and Lip Gloss. Elizabeth Arden's "Lip Spa" uses a method adapted from a scientist at Uniliver, its conglomerate parent company, that emulsifies chocolate to reinvent lipstick.

- **Chocolate Memo Pads** are available through Once Upon a Planet in Bayside, New York.

- Sandra Katzman of Confections by Sandra in Canoga Park, California, created a chocolate **Monopoly** game that sold through the Neiman-Marcus catalogue in 1978 for $600.

- **Music** lovers who also happen to be chocolate lovers can have songs in their hearts with mugs decorated with notes, instruments, lyrics, etc.–filled with chocolate, then refilled with hot chocolate.

- Harry and David of Medford, Oregon, offer "An Unherd-of Valentine Gift"–an actual **Chocolate Moose**, one pound of milk chocolate that they suggest sending to deer friends. Very amoosing.

- Cosmetic Arts and Company of Clark, New Jersey, offers a line of "Chocolate Creams" **nail polish**.

- **Nightshirts** are available through ABEL-express of Carnegie, Pennsylvania, with these sayings: 1. "Do not disturb–CHOCOLATE FANTASY in progress"; 2. "Promise me anything but give me CHOCOLATIER."

- Sweetvisions Publishing Company of Newton Highlands, Massachusetts, has put out some luscious **notecards** with pictures of chocolate photographed by Robert Kaufman in their "Sweetness and Light" series.

- Cocoa Notes puts out chocolate-colored and scented **notepads**, printed with sweet slogans.

- Design, Inc. of Farmingdale, New York, made a special line of chocolate **New York City subway tokens** for Macy's.

- Sweet **Chocolate Peppers** have been developed by the University of New Hampshire that supposedly ripen just 58 days after transplanting.

- If **pistachios** are your passion, you can get a pound of them, chocolate-covered, from P.O. Box 51590 in Pacific Grove, California.

- The Great American Puzzle Factory of New York has 550-piece **puzzles** of "Hershey Kisses" and "Hershey's Assorted Miniatures."

- S. E. Rykoff and Company of Los Angeles offers a box of 120 **Reception Sticks** for demitasse: orange, lemon, mint, and cinnamon-flavored spun sugar dipped in bittersweet chocolate.

- Motta Chocolates of Italy produces **replicas** of chocolate ravioli, seafood, and ice cream cones.

- **Risk Enterprises** of Cleveland, a graphic design group owned by Brian Fenderbosch, has produced a number of chocolate-related novelties such as aprons, painter's caps, T-shirts, and more.

- In the United States, "adult chocolate" usually refers to chocolate shaped like **sexual organs**; its counterpart in Europe might be a heavily liqueored chocolate bar.

- Barcelona confectioner Jose Balceela Pallares and his assistant Xavier Salvat created an 8-1/2-foot, 229-lb semisweet chocolate sculpture of the **Statue of Liberty** in three intensive days of work. For the July 4th, 1986, Statue of Liberty Centennial, master chocolatier Paul Berthon of Paris created a 14-foot, 4,000-pound pure bittersweet chocolate replica. Made using an original mold from the Louvre, the statue contained an estimated $30,000 worth of chocolate, and took Chef Berthon and two assistants 800 hours to create.

- The **Swiss Colony** of Monroe, Wisconsin, has many interesting chocolate cakes, tortes, petit fours, and novelty chocolates, such as Santa's Helpers, gingerbread houses, chocolate "records," chocolate roses, chocolate cordials, plus Chipolate Chocolate Chunks, Fudge Holiday Kisses, giant chocolate cups, and chocolate mint sticks at Christmastime.

- Recycled Paper Products of Chicago has a **T-shirt** with a Boynton design bearing this message: "EMERGENCY ALERT. If wearer of this shirt is found vacant, listless, or depressed, AD-MINISTER CHOCOLATE IMMEDIATELY." Dallas Alice, out of Rockville, Maryland, has T-shirts proclaiming "Open Mouth, Insert Chocolate," "Chocolate Spoken Here," "Save the Chocolate Mousse," "Know Your Chocolate Bar," and others. Hawk Enterprise of San Francisco features a "Save the Chocolate Mousse" T-shirt, while Leonard Agnello has one that reads "Stamp out herpes–give chocolate kisses." Sweets, Inc. in Brooklyn has a T-shirt that says, "The Lord loveth a chocolate giver."

- Cutter Bill's of Dallas produces **"A Taste of Texas,"** a bas-relief of the state in chocolate.

- Any number of these items can be ordered by your own chocolate **telephone**.

- St. Moritz Luxury Chocolates of Beverly Hills offers a chocolate **tennis racquet** accompanied by a box of eight truffles–for the consolations, perhaps?

- A chocolate **"Thank You Medallion"** is available from Geneve Chocolatier of Madison, Wisconsin. The 8-1/2", 12-oz floral medallion, made of pure milk chocolate, offers thanks in four languages: English, French, German, and Spanish.

- The Smoke Scene, Inc. in New York City sells "Chocolate cake chocolate burley" **tobacco.**

- **Tobler** makes a book of chocolates that has a reusable cover, jewelry boxes with three drawers of chocolates, mechanized boxes of Berne chocolate bears or racing cars, and miniature assortments with scenic vistas of Switzerland.

- If you dream of a world of chocolate, **Topographic Chocolates** has reproductions of the Grand Canyon, Yosemite National Park, the Matterhorn, Pebble Beach Golf Course, Squaw Valley, etc. Where there are mountains, such as at Mount Everest, white chocolate is used over the company's Guittard milk chocolate for snow-capped peaks.

- Dilettante Chocolates of Seattle makes a number of terrific **toppings**, such as Dilettante Ephemera Sauce, Dilettante Truffle Topping, Carameled Cream Ice Cream Topping, and Dilettante Chocolate Fondue.

- **Transportation** is the key to Harry C. Nagel & Sons novelties. The West New York, New Jersey, firm fills orders for chocolate airplanes, trains, cars, or whatever you request.

- Sweet Investments, Inc. of Goleta, California offers **"The Ultimate Sweet Tooth,"** a 1-lb molar crafted in pure milk chocolate. Created by a California dentist, John Elissen, the tooth sells for about $10.

- Andre Bollier Ltd. produces a life-size chocolate **wine bottle** filled with 10 ounces of California raisins.

- Trifles includes an 8″, 16-oz solid milk chocolate **wreath** under its mail-order suggestions for the holidays.

Chapter III

Chocolate Folklore

CHOCOLATE COMPANIES

- **Akutagawa Confectionery** of Japan makes a number of chocolate novelty items in addition to its "Piaffer" chocolate wafers.

- **Ambrosia Chocolate** of Milwaukee began in 1894 by making consumer-oriented treats, but today it manufactures bulk chocolate in 10-lb cakes and 23-ton liquid chocolate in tanks. Its products are familiar to you in the form of Hostess Cupcakes, Heath Bars, Dolly Madison Cupcakes, and Eskimo Pies; when you purchase products made by Keebler, Pillsbury, Nabisco, Quaker Oats, or Swiss Miss, you're consuming Ambrosia. A division of W. R. Grace and Company since 1964, it is the largest industrial supplier of chocolate and confectionery products to the world.

- "Chocolate as you've never known it before" is available from the **Astor Chocolate Corporation**, headquartered at 48-25 Metropolitan Avenue in Glendale, New York 11385 (718/386-7400). It offers a number of chocolate novelties, including a solid chocolate chess set, chocolate dessert shells, chocolate hazelnut truffles, and a number of different chocolate cards for every occasion.

- A part of General Foods since 1927, **Walter Baker & Co., Inc.** began as a cocoa and chocolate enterprise in 1765 "on the bank of the Neponset River at Dorchester, where it falls to tidewater in Boston Harbor." It was the first chocolate mill in America. Beginning in 1872, it used as its symbol "Le Belle Chocolatiere," a

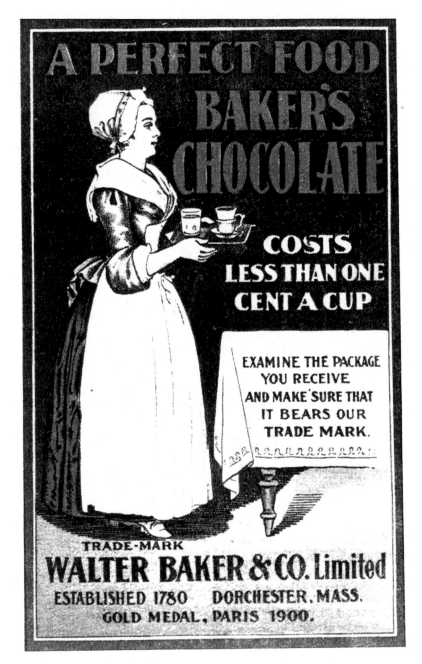

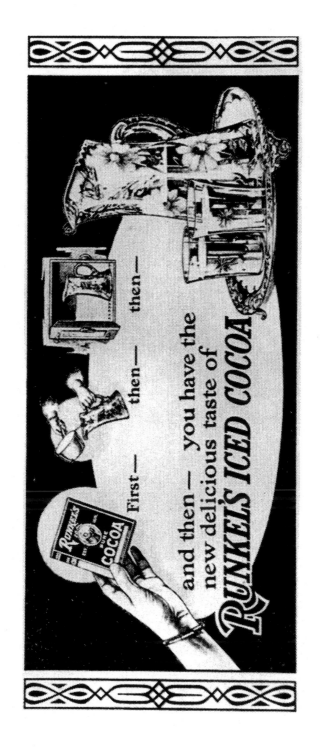

First — then — then —

and then — you have the new delicious taste of RUNKEL'S ICED COCOA painting inspired when Ditrichstein, a Prince of the realm, fell in love with a waitress (Anna Baltauf, the daughter of knight Melchior Baltauf) who served him chocolate in Vienna in 1760. They were betrothed, and Ditrichstein engaged the talented Swiss painter Jean Etienne Leotard to paint his fiancée in costume as he first saw her. Today the portrait hangs in the Dresden Gallery.

- While they are made with cocoa, the ingredient that makes chocolate really chocolate, **Barat Chocolates** (201/882-9190) use substitutes for other ingredients: instead of refined white sugar, they use Sucanat–organic granulated cane juice that is high in vitamins, calcium, and iron; further, they use tofu instead of dairy products.

- Famous for its fabulous "Chocolate Catalogue," **Karl Bissinger** French Confections of St. Louis has packaged its boxes since 1863 with the seal of its founder as "Confiseur Imperial" to French Emperor Louis Napoleon.

- **Blommer Chocolate Company** of East Greenfield, Pennsylvania, is one of the five largest manufacturers of industrial or bulk chocolate in the United States. Started by the three Blommer brothers in 1939, Blommer today uses about 100 million pounds of chocolate per year. According to Martin E. Krueger, Vice President, it manufactures "a wide range of chocolate and confectionery coatings" in the company's three plants.

- Holidays are featured events at **Sydney Bogg Chocolates** in Detroit, where owners Ralph and Doris Skidmore produce items such as chocolate Irish potatoes for St. Patrick's Day, chocolate and caramel apples at Halloween, and Sweetheart Assortments at Valentine's Day. The company began in 1936, and Mr. Skidmore declares that whenever he says anything to the media, he always prefaces it by saying, "Chocolate is the world's favorite flavor."

- **Boldemann Chocolate Company** dates back to the 1880s, when the Union City, California, firm was looking for a bulk product–since freight was such an expensive item and they wanted to get the best shipping rate. The Boldemann family chose chocolate, and today it's one of the biggest chocolate manufacturers in the United States.

- **E. J. Brach & Sons** of Chicago was founded in 1904, then merged with American Home Products in 1966. The company's Senior Vice President for Sales and Marketing assures us that "chocolates are an important and growing section of our confectionery business." The company's slogan is: "Nobody treats America like Brach's."

- **Cadbury's** "Factory in a Garden" dates from 1830, when John Cadbury introduced cocoa powder to his coffee and tea shop in Birmingham, England. Its milk to this day is pure dairy milk, not the usual skimmed, dried milk used by many chocolate manufacturers. The world's largest chocolate producer, Cadbury's has factories worldwide. Peter Paul Cadbury, Inc. is a member of the Cadbury-Schweppes Group.

- A handmade product since 1911, **Chardon Chocolates** of Zurich are now flown weekly to New York City via Swiss Air. They are available at 24 East 66th Street, NY.

- Members of the **Chocolate Manufacturers Association of the U.S.A.** include: Ambrosia Chocolate Company, The Blommer Chocolate Company, E. J. Brach & Sons, Cocoline Chocolate Company, Inc., Ghirardelli Chocolate Company, Guittard Chocolate Company, L. S. Heath & Sons., Inc., Hershey Foods Corporation, Hooton Chocolate Company, Luden's, Inc., M&M/Mars, Inc., The Nestle Company, Peter Paul Cadbury, Inc., Van Leer Chocolate Corporation, and World's Finest Chocolate, Inc.

- "We are among the nation's first chocolate bakeries . . . and we are the best," says **Cocolat** of Berkeley, California. Founded in 1976, it is run by Alice and Elliott Medrich.

- **Cocoline Chocolate Company** in Brooklyn manufactures chocolate from basic raw material: cocoa beans, sugar, milk, etc. Joseph Kaufman, Director of Marketing, says, "Chocolate manufacturing is our business."

- **Chocolaterie H. Corne de la Toison d'Or** of Belgium bases its motto, "No other shall I have," on a 15th century legend about King Philip the Good of France, who created an order of chivalry based on virtue; his creed was "Aultre Nautray." The company celebrated its centennial in 1983 with "une soiree de gala exceptionnelle."

- Gary Goldberg of the **Culinary Center of New York** talks about their chocolate offerings: (1) chocolate weekends for courses with Martin Johner, "The Chocolate Chef"; (2) a 40-minute film entitled "Chocolate" that is available for VCRs; (3) "Tres Chocolat" ice cream that it supplies to restaurants. Goldberg spouts a fun philosophy: "A good dessert has no more calories than a small one."

- **Debauve and Gallais** Chocolate Shop in Paris emerged in the mid-nineteenth century from the cojoining of a pharmacy (Monsieur Gallais) and a chocolatier (Monsieur Debauve), who originally sold their chocolate mixtures as panaceas.

- Formulas for **Dilettante Chocolates** of Seattle have been handed down from pastry chef Julius Rudolf Franzen of Budapest, master candy maker, to Czar Nicholas II of Russia, to a third generation of chocolatiers, the Davenport family. Formulated to give "more flavor than sweetness," Dilettante chocolates has won national awards and recognition for its sauces, toppings, and chocolate dragees.

- Famous for its chocolate pâté, **Double Truffle** of Beverly Hills is a classic case of a cottage industry that has become an industry leader. Roman DeValenti, the owner, commented that chocolate is a very volatile product, and that Double Truffle aims at a very selective target niche.

- **Elite Chocolates** of Israel produces kosher chocolates, cocoa, and chocolate-coated halva. Their candy bars were a pleasant surprise to me in Jerusalem, given the warm summer temperatures.

- **Fanny Farmer** Candy Shops, named for the first American to put her recipes into a cookbook, began operation in 1919. Today Fanny Farmer has more than 350 stores in 22 states.

- "Control production" is the key to **Fannie May's** Chicago candies, started by H. Teller Archibald in 1920. A daily inventory is kept so that any candy not sold in two weeks is removed from the shelves. Fannie May's chocolate-covered cherries and bonbons are still hand-dipped.

- Founded in 1908, **Max Felchlin's** "Fabrik fur die Konditorei" of Schwyz, Switzerland, specializes in the manufacture of chocolate, bakery products, and special creams. In addition, it operates six sensational restaurant/candy shops under the name of "Vanini." Bakers, chefs, and confectioners throughout Europe, the United States, and Japan appreciate the high quality and commitment to consistency found in Max Felchlin products.

- **J & A Ferguson's** Scottish firm features a "Nine Reigns" box assortment of chocolates that celebrates the British monarchs who have reigned during its more than a century of operation—from King George III to Queen Elizabeth II.

- An international business, with multimillion-dollar sales, more than 400 domestic stores and many others around the world, **Mrs. Fields** uses 10% of the world's macadamia crop.

- Operating like an art gallery, **Galerie Au Chocolat** shops (in New York, Palm Beach, Phoenix, Pittsburgh, Cincinnati, and Annapolis) allow customers to select chocolates individually from more than 100 choices.

- Site of the old **Ghiardelli** chocolate factory, Ghiardelli Square in San Francisco was renovated in 1964 by shipping heiress Lurline M. Roth to sell ice cream, ground chocolate and cocoa, baking chocolate, and various novelty items. Established in 1852, Ghiardelli became a division of the Golden Grain Macaroni Company in 1962.

- **Gianduia,** acclaimed by some as the finest chocolate in the world, is dealt with through the Italian Institute for Foreign

Trade. For their "History of the Pasticceria," contact the Italian Trade Commission at 499 Park Avenue, New York, New York 10022 (212/980-1500).

- The Belgian company **Godiva Chocolatier, Inc.** has been owned by the Campbell Soup Company since 1966. All of its chocolates are shell-molded, then exquisitely packaged in a gold "Ballotin" (box). Although Godiva's Belgian chocolates are predominantly illegal for importation because of their liquor content, the chocolates produced here dominate 50% of the luxury chocolate market in the United States. Godiva Chocolatier, Inc. has an advertising budget of nearly a half-million dollars and has seen a 400+% increase in sales since 1979.

- In 1944 **Bill and Helen Grace** opened a candy shop in San Pedro "with a smile and confections that pleased our customers." Today, Helen Grace Chocolates (800/367-4240) is headquartered at 3303 Century Boulevard in Lynwood, California, having added more than a dozen shops and having expanded to about 100 chocolate specialties. Three generations of the Grace family are continuing the tradition.

- **Grand Finale** of Berkeley, which bills itself as "California's smallest licensed candy factory," puts out a two-page "non-lavish catalogue" showing its buttercream caramels, dessert sauces, and triple-chocolate truffles.

- Master Chef **Michel Guerard** uses 25% less sugar than is customarily used in chocolate-making. In an advertisement for Michel Guerard, "La Cuisine Chocolat Imported from Belgium," one is guided in determining fine quality chocolate by three aspects: taste (dark chocolate should be floral, aromatic; milk chocolate should have a subtle, nutty flavor), bouquet, and texture (extraordinarily smooth, melting evenly and quickly in your mouth).

- **Guittard Chocolate Company** in Burlingame, California, was founded in 1868 by Etienne Guittard, and the company has remained a family business for four generations. A major chocolate producer, Guittard supplies confectionery, baking, and ice cream customers throughout the United States and the world. Try to visit them–there's a cocoa tree growing in the lobby.

- What began as a hobby in 1973 in Ben Strohecker's Marblehead, Massachusetts, kitchen to "make the best candy in the world, regardless of cost," is the happy result today of **Harbor Sweets, Inc.** Although best known for its nautical themes like Sweep Sloops, Marblehead Mints, and Sand Dollars, Harbor Sweets does special fund-raising orders for museums, clubs, and civic and cultural organizations.

- **Hauser Chocolatier** in Bethel, Connecticut, offers Swiss-style truffles "for the discriminating chocolate connoisseur." Hauser has a number of clever animal-shaped chocolates, such as pandas, bunnies, chickens, pigs, and ducks.

- Billing itself as "Makers of America's Finest Candy Bar," **L. S. Heath & Sons, Inc.** began in Robinson, Illinois, in 1914. From a series of trial-and-error experiments, "English Toffee" was concocted in 1928. The sons discovered a clever way to get the toffee marketed: they included a check-box on Heath's home-delivery dairy forms for "Heath English Toffee Bars"; its popularity remains legend. The product was introduced into the marketplace nationwide in 1958. L. S. Heath today is still a privately held corporation, with stock owned solely by members of the Heath family.

- With headquarters in Shrewsbury, Massachusetts, the **Hebert Candy Mansion** is where "ivory candy" (white chocolate) was discovered as a way of allowing people to enjoy chocolate during the warm summer months. A retail manufacturer since 1917, Hebert is a multimillion-dollar industry today, producing over 400 items. Its motto is: "Remember that New England is famous for the best candy in the world, and that Hebert Candies is famous for the best candy in New England."

- **Hershey Foods Corporation** of Hershey, Pennsylvania, with annual sales of $2+ billion, is *the* chocolate giant. Hershey Foods is the foremost researcher on the chemistry of the cocoa bean, mainly through its experimental cacao tree farm in the Central American country of Belize. Along with M&M/Mars, the two corporations control nearly 70% of the candy market. Hershey Foods' advertising budget is around one quarter of a million dollars. According to Jay F. Carr, Vice President of Marketing, Hershey's products include bar goods, bagged items, baking ingredients, chocolate drink mixes, and dessert toppings. Visitors to Hershey headquarters get to tour Zoo America, Hershey Museum of American Life, Hershey Gardens, Chocolate World (a free tour of the manufacturing process that produces "The Great American Chocolate Bar"), Founders Hall, and Hershey Park.

- **Hofbauer Vienna, Ltd.** has been using the official crest of the Austrian government on its packages since 1882.

- "California's Finest Chocolates," **Hooper's Chocolates** of Oakland has been a family tradition for three generations, since 1939.

- **Hooton Chocolate Company** of Newark, New Jersey, was established in 1897, and is now a division of W. R. Grace & Co. Hooton's logo is an owl, proclaiming it "the smart choice."

- "Tempting to the eye, Irresistible to the palate!"–**Huwyler** of Switzerland flies its freshly made truffles each week to New York and Chicago via SwissAir.

- **Imports Unlimited** of Peterborough, New Hampshire, offers "douceurs de france," delicious French chocolate delicacies that come packaged in an elegant lace sac.

- When they bill themselves as **Jerbeau Handmade Chocolates**, the Los Angeles-based company means that they hand-roll, hand-dip, and hand-pack all their chocolates. As a final touch, each box is printed with a child's chocolate handprint.

- **Kosher Chocolate Factory** in Northfield, Illinois, offers purely natural, "pareve" products, made with no milk, animal products, preservatives, or extenders. Under the supervision of the Chicago

Rabbinical Council, their chocolates contain sugar, chocolate liquor, cocoa butter, soya lecithin, and vanilla.

- **Josip Kras**, one of the oldest chocolate companies in Yugoslavia, mostly sells prepackaged chocolates for other companies.

- Hungarian-trained chocolatier **Tom Kron** of New York City likes to mold chocolate into amusing shapes, sometimes then filling them with fruits and nuts. All chocolate is made in Kron's New York factory, but each one of its chocolate shops dips its own fruit each day.

- With 280 shops, **Leonidas/D'Orsay** is Belgium's largest chocolate producer.

- **Liled's Candy Kitchen**, a Vallejo tradition since Halloween day of 1936, uses Guittard's Old Dutch coating for its milk chocolate, nuts from India, Pakistan, and Bolivia, coffee from Africa and South America, coconut from the Philippines, and cream, eggs, butter, almonds, walnuts, and choice fruits from its own California.

- Swiss technology is the key to success for the "**Lindt and Sprungli** Chocolate Process" (LSCP), which examines all cocoa beans by means of chromatography, tests all sugar, and uses a "rancidity meter" on all its nuts. The tradition dates to 1845, when master confectioner Rudolf Sprungli first produced chocolate. The company became Lindt & Sprungli in 1899, developing subsidiaries in Berlin (1928) and England (1932), and license agreements with Italy (1946), Germany (1950), and France (1954). The company has continually grown and developed new methods of excellence and efficiency. For example, its 1979 Elegance Box features "the softest, most fragile truffled chocolates imaginable." When Lindt chocolate started being used in David's Cookies that same year, sales skyrocketed. Today, Lindt & Sprungli produces 50 tons of chocolate per day, more than 20 million pounds per year, for more than 500 chocolate products. The company's work is based on five pillars:

1. The determination to remain independent;
2. The endeavor to realize an ample profit;
3. The resolution to be active in the top quality range only;
4. The intention to guide the enterprise according to active, dynamic, and, at the same time, traditional principles;
5. The resolution to act according to ethical fundamental rules.

- Trained in Switzerland, **Lisa Lerner Chocolatier** of Berkeley has developed a "California truffle" that is larger than usual and contains different, innovative flavors. Several different gift plans are available.

- **Harry London's** Gourmet Chocolates of North Canton, Ohio, produces a number of humorous chocolate novelty items, such as Super Kiss, chocolate pacifiers, chocolate Bingo cards, milk chocolate footballs, a chocolate "get well" pill, and many, many more. Founded in 1922, Harry London has annual sales of more than $7 million.

- From a small local candy manufacturer in Reading, Pennsylvania, in 1881, **Luden's, Inc.** has been a privately held corporation most famous for its cough drops but also for its chocolate Fifth Avenue Bars, Mellomint Patties, hollow chocolate, and novelties.

- The name for Belgium's **Chocolatier Manon** of New York City derives from that of a legendary dairy maid, Manon Lescault. The company's classic antique molds have been used since 1910, forming the light and dark chocolates filled with praline, butter cream, and creme fraiche.

- **"Madame Chocolate"** is really the talented and personable Elaine Sherman, author of *Madame Chocolate's Book of Divine Indulgences* (Contemporary Books, 1984). In what she labels a "Mom-Pop Operation" out of Glenview, Illinois, Madame Chocolate has a mailing list of 40,000 for her mail-order catalogue, which welcomes them with the statement, "As a chocoholic, I strive to bring to you the very finest chocolate–foreign and domestic–for cooking, baking, and candy-making." Some of her offerings include Sweet Treats, Deep Dark Secrets, Bittersweet Experience, Essential Extras, Main Line, Light Line, Big Blondes, Sweet Harmony, Great Pretenders, Bit & Pieces, Cocoa Connection, and many more.

- Family-owned and operated since 1882, **Moreau Chocolates** of Switzerland depends on a number of international sources for its products: cocoa beans from Venezuela and Central America, hazelnuts from Italy, almonds from California, and fresh cream from its own nearby Jura Mountains.

- A subsidiary of Nabisco, **Merckens Chocolate Company** makes the cocoa for Oreo cookies, the chocolate drops in Chips Ahoy, and the coating for Sugar Daddies. Housed in a chocolate factory in Mansfield, Massachusetts, that dates back to 1903, it operates by a process in which cocoa beans are delivered to the top floor, then are processed floor by floor on downward until they become chocolate.

- **The Nestle Company, Inc.** began in Switzerland in 1866 when Henri Nestle formulated a unique milk product for infants. Chocolate manufacturer Daniel Peter used Nestle's invention to produce the world's first milk chocolate in 1875, and by 1900 the company opened its first manufacturing facility in the United States. The Nestle Crunch Bar was developed in 1938, followed soon by Toll House Morsels, ChocoLite, Hot Cocoa Mix, Quik, $100,000 Bar, Go Ahead, Crunch Ice Cream Bar, the Nestle Chocolate Chip Sandwich, etc. Today, the Nestle Company is the world's largest food corporation, cornering about 10% of the American chocolate market.

- **Neuhaus,** recognized as one of the leading imported luxury chocolates, is mostly sold in exclusive department stores. A Belgian specialty since 1851, Neuhaus USA began operation in 1981 out of Rego Park, New York. Today the chocolates are handcrafted and made the same way they originally were. There are more than 100 varieties available. Two manufacturing processes are used: some chocolates are made inside out, where centers (nuts, toffee, marzipan) are wrapped in chocolate; others are molded chocolate cups, filled with creme fraiche, praline, or liquor extract. Neuhaus has annual sales of about $2 million.

- Legend has it that a particular line of handmade chocolates got a rating that gave **Osogud Candies** of Pasadena, California, its name.

- **Neuchatel Chocolates** fly their bulk chocolate in weekly from Switzerland to New York, then have it molded into candy shapes.

- Pepino Buitoni began manufacturing chocolates in 1907, and decided to name them for his Italian locality: **Perugina**. Introduced to the United States at the 1939 World's Fair, Perugina makes chocolate with distinct names, histories, and packaging. Their catalogue announces how Perugina chocolate is unique: "An irresistible combination of African and South American cocoa. Made always with natural cocoa butter. Use only the 'best in crop,' the choicest hazelnuts, almonds, and cherries from the best Italian harvests."

- Founded in 1848, **Poulain Chocolat Confiserie** has been owned since 1980 by Sanofi, a French pharmaceutical subsidiary of Elf Aquitaine. With a 17% share of the French chocolate bar market and 23% of the French chocolate drink market, it also makes chocolate confectionery and industrial chocolate out of its manufacturing plant in Blois, France. 1983 sales were $79 million.

- "Kentucky Colonels," made of 100-proof bourbon, are **Rebecca-Ruth's** fantastic concoction; they are only available in Kentucky, where they are legal. The company was formed in 1919 by Ruth Booe, mother of the current president, John C. Booe, and her friend Rebecca Gooch.

- **Red Tulip Chocolates Pty, Ltd.** of Victoria, Australia, have been "Makers of Fine Chocolates" since 1953. They offer a range of over 1,000 products, split evenly between sugar and chocolate. The Australian company is owned by Beatrice Foods of Chicago.

- In the Elliott Family for more than 55 years, **Regina's Fine Chocolates** of St. Paul, Minnesota, uses as its slogan "A Complete Chocolate Experience." Now a third-generation company, Regina's includes in its brochure, "A Candyland Fantasy with Over 400 Varieties," the following history: "Regina's Candy Shops are a family affair, a legacy from a young Greek craftsman and his bride, Regina, to their children and grandchildren."

- "The peak of perfection in handmade chocolates" is what **The Rocky Mountain Chocolate Factory** of Durango, Colorado, calls itself. Founded in 1981, already it is a $10 million corporation, involved in manufacturing, wholesaling, franchising, and distributing its own products to 40 stores in nine states, and anticipating wide expansion in the future. Frank Crail, founder and president, shared the following with *Entrepreneur* magazine (April 1985, p. 68): "You make your own success. You do your research, analyze the market, take a calculated risk, and follow through as thoroughly as possible. It's important to understand your limitations." According to Thomas N. Hansen, Director of Marketing, The Rocky Mountain Chocolate Factory boasts 60 varieties of handmade chocolates, plus six flavors of gourmet chocolate sauce. Many of these items are showcased in a variety of paper and wood packaging.

- **Gladys Ronsvalle** talks enthusiastically about her chocolate-making activities in Syracuse, New York. In business for over 50 years, she is very service-oriented, and ships more than 200 kinds of chocolate all over–especially her famous "Chippies," chocolate-coated potato chips made into patties.

- **The San Francisco Chocolate Company** features a "Marilla" line, boxed and unboxed chocolate, a farmyard series (for example, the pig has a Grand Marnier center dipped pink, the chicken Bailey's Irish Creme center dipped white), animal series, medallions, and pretzels.

- You can get sugarfree taffy and caramels at **Miss Saylor's Candies** in Long Beach, California, in addition to boxed and bulk chocolate.

- **Joseph Schmidt Confections** of San Francisco (415/861-8682) was created in 1983 by partners Audrey Ryan and Joseph Schmidt. It has been honored by national art shows for its delicate hand-painted chocolate sculptures, and counts many famous clients around the world.

- Senator O'Connor of Toronto had quite a reputation for making quality candy, and when friends suggested he make it into a business, he did. **Laura Secord**, named for the Canadian heroine of the War of 1812, began in 1913. In the mid-1970s, it merged with the Smiles 'n Chuckles Candy Company of Ontario, noted for its "Turtles." One of the largest candy companies in the world, there are more than 210 Laura Secord Candy Shops from coast to coast in Canada. According to Brian K. Harrison, Marketing Manager, the Smiles Confectionery Division sells a variety of branded candy products through more traditional mass-market outlets.

- **See's Candy Shops** of California ships its candy throughout the year and guarantees its quality. Operating out of factories in Los Angeles and San Francisco, See's slogan since 1921 has been "Quality without compromise." Each box features a cameo of Mary See, attesting to the company's enduring tradition. Donald K. Hawley, Administrative Coordinator of Advertising and Public Relations, points out that See's is "most successful, with 218 shops from Hong Kong to Disney World in Florida."

- **Lee Sims Chocolates** are crafted in Jersey City, New Jersey. The company is most famous for its "pyramids," assorted boxes that stack up to look like pyramids.

- Goo Goos are the most famous product of the **Standard Candy Company** of Nashville, TN. The clusters, a concoction of caramel, marshmallow, and peanuts covered with milk chocolate, celebrated their 75th year in 1986. Each bar weighs less than 2 ounces, counts 240 calories, and costs about 50 cents.

- Karl Stork, president-chocolatier of **Stork's Pastry Shop, Inc.** in Whitestone, New York, features "baumkuchen" (a generations-old "Tree Cake," favored by European royalty), "escargots" (chocolate snail shells), marzipan, "cat tongues," and tantalizing truffles.

- **Sucrs. de Pedro Cortes, Inc.** of San Juan, Puerto Rico, makes Spanish-style chocolate "cortes" and chocolate powder "choki." Ms. Norma Sanchez, Director of Marketing, says they use intermediaries such as supermarkets and grocery stores to reach target markets of kids and housewives.

- **Suchard,** which has operated in Neuchatel, Switzerland, since 1824, maintains a museum of chocolate artifacts, posters, and packaging displays. Its founder, Philipp Suchard, built the first mixing machine for chocolate. Suchard is most famous for its Milka and Bittra chocolate bars, but it also makes an instant chocolate drink and a selection of many other confections. The company merged with Chocolat Tobler, Ltd. in 1970; Tobler-Suchard USA is headquartered in Delavan, Wisconsin.

- **Sweet Swiss/European Specialties** of Spokane, Washington, is run by Joe and Edith Nendl. Ingredients for the confections truly are European, including French champagne extract for truffles, Italian amarena cherries for the cordials, Callebaut chocolate couverture from Belgium, and Swiss Kirschwasser for brandy truffles.

- **Joseph Terry & Sons, Ltd.** of York, England, was founded in 1767 for confectioneries, and then its chocolate factory was built in 1886. One of its most famous products is Terry's milk chocolate orange, 20 pieces shaped like an orange.

- For more than half a century, **Teuscher Chocolates** of Zurich have been made without preservatives or additives. Their brightly colored packaging, designed by Felix Daetwyler, is replete with child-like symbols.

- **Chocolate Tobler, Ltd.** has had many different titles since it was founded by Jean Tobler in 1867 in Berne, Switzerland. Establishing its first subsidiary in 1901, Tobler today has them worldwide:

Germany, France, Italy, Spain, England, Austria, Argentina, Brazil; further, it is licensed in Australia, Ireland, Yugoslavia, and Japan. Tobler has been doing business in the United States for two decades. It merged with the Suchard Group in 1970, forming Multifood, Ltd. Tobler-Suchard is a subsidiary of Jacobs Suchard AG of Zurich; it has international sales in more than 100 countries of $2 billion. Tobler-Suchard USA supports skiing events, cooking demonstrations, and sampling at chocolate events.

- **E. A. Tosi and Sons Co., Inc.** of Braintree, Massachusetts, is a chocolate importer who supplies chocolate to institutional suppliers, chefs, hotels, etc. It is a closely held corporation.

- A newcomer to the chocolate industry is **Toucan Chocolates** of 31 Wyman Street, P.O. Box 72, Waban, Massachusetts 02168 (617/964-8696). Part of its proceeds go to Cultural Survival, Inc. for work in helping inhabitants of tropical forest regions. In addition to supporting global human rights, owners Michael and Susan Goldman also demonstrate on local environmental concern, using no plastics in their packaging, 100% recycled paper and stock, and vegetable-based inks.

- Cousins and partners Nancy Cummins and Karen Weber run the highly successful **UAI Productions** of Northridge, California, as a service to the chocolate industry. Their activities have included chocolate cruises, chocolate festivals and events, and chocolate trips and tours.

- The leading manufacturer of dietetic chocolate coatings in the United States is the **Van Leer Chocolate Corporation** of Jersey City, New Jersey. L. K. Van Leer imported Holland Dutch Cocoa Powders in 1930, then began manufacturing chocolate in 1950. The company's most popular products are its milk chocolate, bittersweet and vanilla chocolate compound, dietetic and ice cream bar coatings, cocoa butter and filbert pastes, chocolate liquor, and cocoa powders. Malcolm Campbell, Executive Vice President of Van Leer, says that increasing consumer awareness of quality chocolate is one of the company's main goals.

- Vicki Fioranelli, a former Home Economics teacher, began making chocolates in her home, then decided to form her own shop: **Vicki's Fine Chocolates** of Cleveland, Mississippi. Calling itself "The Sweetest Place in Town," Vicki's features humorous novelty items like a carton of chocolate filled with chocolate buttons, Dolly Lolly, and Santa-face suckers. Vicki has developed a slide presentation which she gives to local clubs and organizations, and encourages field trips to her store. She is one of only two retail confectioners in the whole state, and points out that chocolate is relatively new to the South.

- Those Whitman's Samplers you've always enjoyed got their beginnings when Stephen F. Whitman founded **Whitman's Chocolates** on Market Street in Philadelphia in 1842. Today a manufacturer of boxed chocolate and candy bars, Whitman's is an IC Industries Company, Division of Pet, Inc. It has an advertising budget of $1 million, and encourages consumer feedback. Whitman's recently introduced reduced-calorie "Lite Chocolates," with approximately 40 calories per piece.

- Since 1884, the **Wilbur Chocolate Company** of Lititz, Pennsylvania, has produced chocolate and coatings for many food manufacturers, such as Godiva. A subsidiary of MacAndrews and Forbes, Wilbur produces more than 68 million pounds of chocolate per year for industrial customers, and has annual sales of over $100 million. You may have enjoyed its "Wilbur Buds" and Wilbur Cocoa.

- **C & J Willenborg, Inc.** of Ramsey, New Jersey, is a chocolate importer (of chocolate marzipan, and German and Swiss chocolate) and distributor. Founded in 1927, the company is a subsidiary of Canadian Group, dealing in specialty food products.

- **Williams-Sonoma** of San Francisco has been "Serving Serious Cooks Since 1956." Its chocolate-related products include molds, a glass chocolate thermometer, imported cocoa, couverture chocolate, and hazelnut fudge sauce.

- With no apologies for its name, **World's Finest Chocolate, Inc.** of Chicago was founded in 1922 by Edmond Opler, Sr. Specializing in fund-raising for groups and organizations, it has sold more than two billion chocolate bars since 1957. Besides the Chicago headquarters, World's Finest owns a cocoa plantation in the West Indies and has manufacturing plants in Canada and Australia. Vice President Frank J. Nudd shared videotapes with me that the company has produced about its newly renovated chocolate factory, aimed at being "the most modern and sophisticated in the world." According to Opler, Chairman of the Board, "The world needs more and better chocolate," and World's Finest covers all the bases: making, buying, and selling it. Chocolate, says Opler, is "something everybody loves. You can never get enough chocolate!"

▪ Since 1882, **Milton York Fine Candies** have been produced out of Long Beach, Washington. Those early chocolates were cooked in copper kettles over an open fire, fueled by native alderwood. Milton York bills itself as "the oldest continuous operating candy company in the same location in the country." Today its modern factory produces a wide selection of all-Kosher chocolates.

CHOCOLATE HISTORY

▪ **Confectionery history** has a record of at least 4,000 years, when Egyptians displayed their pleasures on papyrus. Sweetmeats were being sold in the marketplace in 1566 B.C. Yet chocolate didn't appear on the scene until the ancient Aztec and Mayan cultures discovered the value of the cacao plant. It is reputed to have originated in the Amazon or Orinoco basin.

▪ In **600** A.D. the Mayans migrated into the northern regions of South America, establishing the earliest known cocoa plantations in the Yucatan. It has been argued that the Mayans had been familiar with cocoa several centuries prior to this date. They considered it a valuable commodity, used both as a means of payment and as units of calculation.

▪ Mayans and Aztecs took beans from the "cacao" tree and made a drink they called "**xocoatl**." Aztec Indian legend held that cacao

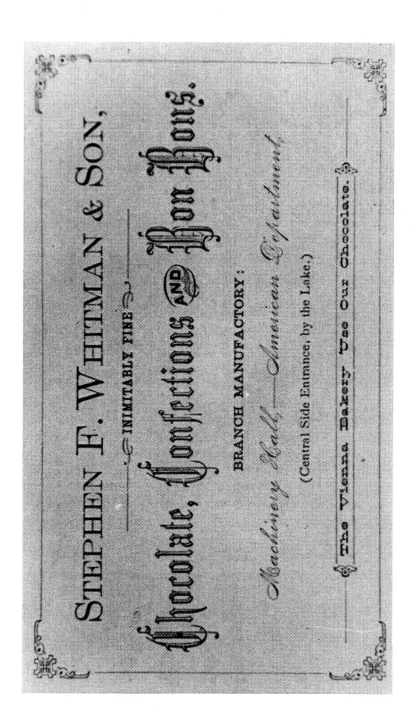

seeds had been brought from Paradise and that wisdom and power came from eating the fruit of the cacao tree.

- Ancient chronicles report that the Aztecs, believing that the god **Quetzalcoatl** travelled to earth on a beam of the Morning Star with a cacao tree from Paradise, took his offering to the people. They learned from Quetzalcoatl how to roast and grind the cacao seeds, making a nourishing paste that could be dissolved in water. They added spices and called this drink "chocolatl," or bitter-water, and believed it brought universal wisdom and knowledge.

- The **word "chocolate"** is said to derive from the Mayan "xocoatl"; cocoa from the Aztec "cacahuatl." The Mexican Indian word "chocolate" comes from a combination of the terms *choco* ("foam") and *atl* ("water"); early chocolate was only consumed in beverage form. As part of a ritual in twelfth-century Mesoamerican marriages, a mug of the frothy chocolate was shared.

- Arthur W. Knapp, author of *The Cocoa and Chocolate Industry* (Pitman, 1923) points out that if we believe **Mexican mythology**, "chocolate was consumed by the Gods in Paradise, and the seed of cocoa was conveyed to man as a special blessing by the God of the Air."

- Ancient Mexicans believed that Tonacatecutli, the goddess of food, and Calchiuhtlucue, the goddess of water, were **guardian goddesses** of cocoa. Each year they performed human sacrifices for the goddesses, giving the victim cocoa at his last meal.

- Swedish naturalist Carolus Linnaeus (1707-1778) was dissatisfied with the word "cocoa," so renamed it **"theobroma,"** Greek for "food of the gods."

- **Christopher Columbus** is said to have brought back cacao beans to King Ferdinand from his fourth visit to the New World, but they were overlooked in favor of the many other treasures he had found.

- Chocolate was first noted in **1519** when Spanish explorer **Hernando Cortez** visited the court of **Emperor Montezuma** of

Mexico. American historian William Hickling's *History of the Conquest of Mexico* (1838) reports that Montezuma "took no other beverage than the *chocolatl*, a potation of chocolate, flavored with vanilla and spices, and so prepared as to be reduced to a froth of the consistency of honey, which gradually dissolved in the mouth and was taken cold." The fact that Montezuma consumed his "chocolatl" in goblets before entering his harem led to the belief that it was an aphrodisiac.

- In 1528 Cortez brought chocolate back from Mexico to the royal court of **King Charles V**. Monks, hidden away in Spanish monasteries, processed the cocoa beans and kept chocolate a secret for nearly a century. It made a profitable industry for Spain, which planted cocoa trees in its overseas colonies.

- It took an Italian traveler, **Antonio Carletti**, to discover the chocolate treasure in 1606 and take it into other parts of Europe.

- "With the decline of Spain as a power, the **secret of cacao** leaked out at last, and the Spanish Crown's monopoly of the chocolate trade came to an end. In a few years the knowledge of it had spread through France, Italy, Germany, and England." (The Nestle Company, Inc., White Plains, New York, *The History of Chocolate and Cocoa*, p. 2.)

- When the Spanish Princess **Maria Theresa** was betrothed to Louis XIV of France in 1615, she gave her fiancé an engagement gift of chocolate, packaged in an elegantly ornate chest. Their marriage was symbolic of the marriage of chocolate in the Spanish-Franco culture.

- The **first chocolate house** was reputedly opened in London in 1657 by a Frenchman. Costing 10 to 15 shillings per pound, chocolate was considered a beverage for the elite class. Sixteenth-century Spanish historian Oviedo noted: "None but the rich and noble could afford to drink chocolatl, as it was literally drinking money. Cocoa passed currency as money among all nations; thus a rabbit in Nicaragua sold for 10 cocoa nibs, and 100 of these seeds could buy a tolerably good slave."

- Chocolate also appears to have been used as a **medicinal remedy** by leading physicians of the day. Christopher Ludwig Hoffmann's treatise *Potus Chocolate* recommends chocolate for many diseases, citing it as a cure for Cardinal Richelieu's ills.

- Chocolate traveled to the **Low Countries** with the Duke of Alba. By 1730, it had dropped in price from $3 per lb to being within the financial reach of those other than the very wealthy. The invention of the cocoa press in 1828 helped further to cut prices and improve the quality of chocolate by squeezing out some of the cocoa butter and giving the beverage a smoother consistency.

- With the **Industrial Revolution** came the mass production of chocolate, spreading its popularity among the citizenry.

- Discussing the introduction of coffee, tea, and cocoa into Europe, Isaac Disraeli (1791-1834) wrote in his six-volume **Curiosities of Literature**: "Chocolate the Spaniards brought from Mexico, where it was denominated *chocolatl*. It was a coarse mixture of ground cacao and Indian corn with roucou; but the Spaniards, liking its nourishment, improved it into a richer compound with sugar, vanilla and other aromatics. We had Chocolate houses in London long after coffee houses; they seemed to have associated something more elegant and refined in their new form when the other had become common."

- **Prince Albert's Exposition** in 1851 in London was the first time the United States was introduced to bonbons, chocolate creams, hand candies (called "boiled sweets"), and caramels.

- An 1891 publication on *The Chocolate-Plant* by Walter Baker & Co. records that, "At the **discovery of America**, the natives of the narrower portion of the continent bordering on the Caribbean Sea were found in possession of two luxuries which have been everywhere recognized as worthy of extensive cultivation; namely, tobacco and chocolate."

- Chocolate was introduced to the United States in 1765 when John Hanan brought cocoa beans from the West Indies into Dorchester, Massachusetts, to refine them with the help of **Dr. James Baker**. The first chocolate factory in the country was established there.

- Yet, chocolate wasn't really accepted by the American colonists until fishermen from Gloucester, Massachusetts, accepted cocoa beans as **payment** for cargo in tropical America.

- Where chocolate was mostly considered a **beverage** for centuries, and predominantly for men, it became recognized as an appropriate drink for children in the seventeenth century. It had many different additions: milk, wine, beer, sweeteners, and spices. Drinking chocolate was considered a very fashionable social event.

- **Eating chocolate** was introduced in 1674 in the form of rolls and cakes, served in the various chocolate emporiums.

- In 1747 Frederick the Great issued an edict forbidding the **hawking of chocolate**.

- By 1795, Dr. Joseph Fry of Bristol, England, employed a steam engine for grinding cocoa beans, an invention that led to the manufacture of chocolate on a **large scale**. Around 1847, Fry & Sons sold a "Chocolat Delicieux a Manger," which is thought to be the first chocolate bar for eating.

- Nestle (*The History of Chocolate and Cocoa*, p. 3) declares that from 1800 to the present day, these four factors contributed to chocolate's **"coming of age"** as a worldwide food product:
  1. The introduction of cocoa powder in 1828;
  2. The reduction of excise duties;
  3. Improvements in transportation facilities, from plantation to factory;
  4. The invention of eating chocolate, and improvements in manufacturing methods.

- By the year 1810, **Venezuela** was producing half the world's requirements for cocoa, and one-third of all the cocoa produced in the world was being consumed by the Spaniards.

- The invention of the **cocoa press** in 1828 by C.J. Van Houten, a Dutch chocolate master, helped reduce the price of chocolate and bring it to the masses. By squeezing out cocoa butter from the beans, Van Houten's "dutching" was an alkalizing process.

- In his 1923 volume *The Cocoa and Chocolate Industry*, Arthur W. Knapp attributes the rise in popularity of cocoa to these **innovations**:

  1. The introduction by Van Houten of cocoa powder as we now know it.
  2. The reduction of the duty to a low figure which remained constant for a number of years.
  3. The great improvements that have taken place in the methods of transport.
  4. Improvements in the manufacture of eating chocolate.

- Daniel Peter of Vevey, Switzerland, experimented for eight years before finally inventing a means of making **milk chocolate** for eating in 1876. He brought his creation to a Swiss firm that today is the world's largest producer of chocolate: Nestle.

- In 1879 Rodolphe Lindt of Berne, Switzerland, produced chocolate that **melted on the tongue**. He invented "conching," a means of heating and rolling chocolate to refine it. After chocolate had been conched for 72 hours and had more cocoa butter added to it, the original "fondant" was created.

- **Cadbury Brothers** displayed eating chocolate in 1849 at an exhibition in Bingley Hall at Birmingham, England.

- Swiss confiseur Jules Sechaud of Montreux introduced a process for manufacturing **filled chocolates** in 1913.

- **The New York Cocoa Exchange**, located at the World Trade Center, was begun October 1, 1925, so that buyers and sellers could get together for transactions.

- Brazil and the Ivory Coast are leaders in the **cocoa bean belt**, accounting for nearly half of the world's cocoa.

- While the United States leads the world in cocoa bean importation and chocolate production, **Switzerland** continues as the leader in per capita chocolate consumption.

- In 1980 a story of **chocolate espionage** hit the world press when an apprentice of the Swiss company of Suchard-Tobler unsuccessfully attempted to sell secret chocolate recipes to Russia, China, Saudi Arabia, and other countries.

- By the 1990s, chocolate had proven its popularity as a product, and its success as a **big business**. Annual world consumption of cocoa beans averages approximately 600,000 tons, and per capita chocolate consumption is greatly on the rise. Chocolate manufacturing in the United States is a multibillion-dollar industry. According to Norman Kolpas (1978, p. 106), "We have seen how chocolate progressed from a primitive drink and food of ancient Latin American tribes–a part of their religious, commerce and social life–to a drink favored by the elite of European society and gradually improved until it was in comparably drinkable and, later, superbly edible. We have also followed its complex transformation from the closely packed seeds of the fruit of an exotic tree to a wide variety of carefully manufactured cocoa and chocolate products. Beyond the historical, agricultural and commercial, and culinary sides to chocolate, others: affect on our health and beauty, and inspiration to literature and the arts."

CHOCOLATE NUTRITION

- The American Medical Association has reported finding no correlation between chocolate and **acne**. And the FDA (Federal Drug Administration) has declared that acne is not diet-related . . . so chocolate can't be blamed.

- Like fine wine, fine chocolate improves with **age**, due to oxidation and chemical interactions. Milk chocolate, however, is best if used within a few months.

- Francois Joseph Victor Broussais (1772-1838) of France, a celebrated physician, proclaimed: "Chocolate of good quality, well made, properly cooked, is one of the best **ailments** that I have yet found for my patients and for myself. This delicious food calms the fever, nourishes adequately the patient, and tends to restore him to health. I would even add that I attribute many cures of chronic dyspepsia to the regular use of chocolate."

- Doctors at the Mayo Clinic report that **allergic reactions** to chocolate are quite rare, and even then are far from life-threatening. Symptoms, when they do occur, vary considerably, but might include itching, hives, and a runny nose.

- W. Hughes, writing in *The American Physician* (1672), called chocolate an **Anodyne** (pain killer), "and exceedingly good to mitigate the pain of gout. . . . It wonderfully refresheth wearied limbs." Chocolate's nutritional value, he felt, "exceeds a Scotchman's provision of Oatmeal and water."

- "**Athletes** have long been aware of the excellent properties of chocolate. Coaches frequently supply their players with chocolate, not only because it boosts energy, but also because it relieves the pangs of hunger some athletes suffer because they eat lightly before an important sports event."

  –Gertrude Parke, 1968

- Beginning in the early seventeenth century, physicians were prescribing chocolate as a **bromide**, a cure-all for their patients.

- The combination of **caffeine and theobromine**, both central nervous system stimulants, gives chocolate its energy-boosting powers. It also helps explain why chocolate has acquired a reputation over the ages of being an aphrodisiac, stimulant, love potion, and magical cure-all. Yet, chocolate's caffeine content has been reported as too slight to stimulate the body, and its theobromine is virtually inactive as a stimulant on the nervous system.

- There are about 5 to 10 milligrams of **caffeine** in one ounce of bittersweet chocolate, 5 milligrams in milk chocolate, and 10 milligrams in a six-ounce cup of cocoa; by contrast, there are 100

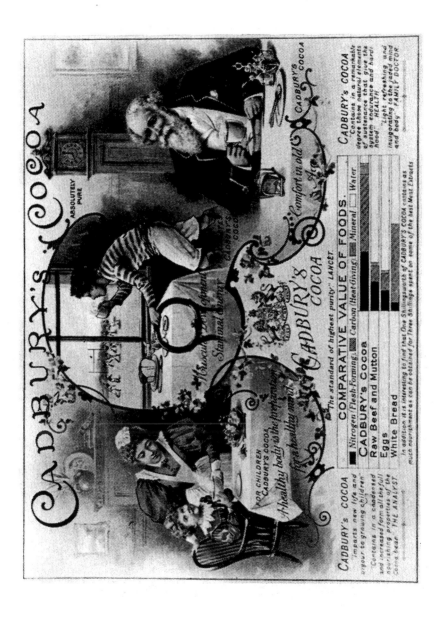

111

to 150 milligrams of caffeine in an eight-ounce cup of brewed coffee. You would have to eat more than a dozen Hershey Bars, for example, to get the amount of caffeine in one cup of coffee.

- The notion that the oxalic acid in chocolate inhibits **calcium absorption** has been disproved by researchers at the University of Illinois, who found statistical insignificance in calcium absorption between persons who included cocoa in their diets and those who ate no cocoa. It is believed that only about 6 our of 250 milligrams of calcium in a cup of chocolate milk is "tied up" as calcium oxalate. Also, a study at the University of Rhode Island found that adding two to three tablespoons of cocoa to 8 ounces of milk significantly reduced bloating and cramps in 37 lactose-intolerant individuals.

- **Calorically**, an apple has about 100 calories; an ounce of chocolate has 150. *The University of Berkeley Wellness Letter* (December 1991) sampled these cocoas and chocolate drinks:

Product	Calories	Fat (g)
Carnation or Nestle hot cocoa	110	1
Swiss Miss Lite hot cocoa	70	-1
Weight Watchers hot cocoa	60	0
Hershey's dry cocoa (1T.)	18	-1
Ghiradelli cocoa	15	1
Nestle Quick drink (2 t.)	72	1
Bosco syrup (2 T.)	85	-1

- Proctor & Gamble has recently applied for FDA approval of a low-calorie fat substitute called **caprenin** for use in confectionery products, since it has characteristics of cocoa butter.

- Cocoa, semi-sweet, and baking chocolate are vegetable-based products, therefore they contain no **cholesterol**. Milk chocolate has a small amount of cholesterol because of its milk content.

- "Although the theobromine of cocoa is now known to be identical with theine and caffeine, the **composition of cocoa** removes it widely from tea and coffee. The quantity of fat varies even in the same sort of cocoa. The ash contains a large quantity of phosphate of potash. The larger quantity of fat makes it a very nourishing article of diet, and it is therefore useful in weak states of the system, and for healthy men under circumstances of great exertion."

–Dr. Edmund A. Parkes, *Manual of Practical Hygiene, prepared especially for use in the Medical Service of the Army* (London, 1864)

- Hubert Howe Bancroft's five-volume *Native Races of the Pacific States of North America* (1875-6) documented that the Aztecs "dug up the bones of giants at the foot of the mountains, and collected by their dwarfish successors, ground to powder, mixed with cocoa, and drank as a **cure for diarrhea and dysentery.**"

- More than 200 sugar-free chocolate desserts are available in Mary Jane Finesand's *The Diabetic Chocolate Cookbook* (Publishers Choice, 1985): candy, cookies, brownies, cakes, cream puffs and eclairs, pudding, pie, even sugar-free chocolate ice cream.

- Chocolate is a complex substance of more than **300 identified compounds**.

- Jane Brody, Personal Health columnist for *The New York Times*, discusses the **decay-inhibiting** property that has been found in chocolate: "When chocolate was added to an otherwise decay-producing diet fed to experimental animals, the incidence of tooth decay dropped. And a study in people at the Forsyth Dental Center in Boston showed that chocolate liquor, when mixed with sucrose, neutralized the effect of sucrose on decay-causing bacteria and interfered with their ability to produce acids from the sugar."

–*Jane Brody's Nutrition Book*, W.W. Norton, 1981

- Christopher Ludwig Hoffman wrote a seventeenth century treatise entitled *Potus Chocolate* that recommended its use in treating many **diseases**, citing the case of Cardinal Richelieu, who was cured of general atrophy by its use.

- Chocolate has long been heralded for its value as an **energy source**. Think of it this way: a single chocolate chip provides sufficient food energy for an adult to walk 150 feet; hence, it would take about 35 chocolate chips to go a mile, or 875,000 for an around-the-world hike.

- Norwegian Arctic explorer Dr. Fridtjob Nansen (1861-1930) records in his book *The First Crossing of Greenland* that chocolate was a critical part of the **equipment:** "We generally used chocolate in the morning . . . (it) is mild in its effect and at the same time nourishing."

- While solid chocolate certainly is high in **fat**, just over half the calories in bittersweet, semisweet, and milk chocolate comes from fat. And even though the cocoa butter in chocolate is mostly saturated fat, studies have shown that it doesn't appear to raise blood cholesterol.

- "The British Government have always believed in cacao for the Navy, and in the early years of the 19th century the amount taken by the Navy formed the mainstay of British consumption . . . the British sailor to this day is given the old-fashioned chocolate, and excellent **fortification** it gives him against the salt breezes."

  –Knapp, *The Cocoa and Chocolate Industry*, 1923.

- The distinguished German physician Christoph Wilhelm Hufeland (1762-1836) recommended "**good chocolate** to nervous, excitable persons; also to the weak, debilitated, and infirm; to children and women. I have obtained excellent results from it in many cases of chronic diseases of the digestive organs."

- "A one-pound package of Runkel's cocoa will supply your body with as much **heat, energy, and walking power** (fuel or calorie value, it is sometimes called) as you can get from five pounds of potatoes, four pounds of fish, three and a half pounds of lean round steak, two one-pound loaves of bread or one and a half pounds of oatmeal." (Runkel's Cocoa Cookery, Est. 1870)

- Samuel Pepys (1633-1703), English Naval officer and diarist, wrote an entry on the chocolate fad in London as a good hangover use for **"imbecility of the stomach."**

- Ten percent of the U.S. Recommended Daily Allowance of **iron** is found in one ounce of baking chocolate or cocoa.

- In a letter to John Adams in 1785, **Thomas Jefferson** made a declaration about chocolate's superiority over tea or coffee for both health and nourishment.

- **Lecithin** is an emulsifier used to reduce the viscosity of chocolate. It serves to lessen the amount of cocoa butter required in the manufacturing process.

- Pamela Hand, an instructor in the veterinary medicine outpatient clinic at Ohio State University, warns that chocolate can be **lethal to dogs**. Theobromine, an ingredient that stimulates the cardiac muscle and the central nervous system, causes chocolate's toxicity. About two ounces of milk chocolate can be poisonous for a 10-lb puppy.

- A 1.5-oz **milk chocolate bar** contains the following nutritive values: protein–6 grams; vitamin A–2.4; trace of vitamin C; thiamine–1.9; riboflavin–9; niacin–.75; calcium–9; iron–3; carbohydrates–24; fat–13.5. If peanuts are added, calories go to 231, protein up to 9 grams.

- It is reported that **Napoleon** carried chocolate with him on his military campaigns, and always ate it when he needed quick energy.

- Dr. Karl Ernest Bock of Leipsig wrote in his "Traite de Pathologie et de Diagnostic": "The nervousness and peevishness of our times are chiefly attributable to tea and coffee. . . . Cocoa and chocolate are **neutral** in their physical effects, and are really the most harmless of our fashionable drinks."

- Chocolate contains certain essential **nutrients**, such as: protein, carbohydrates, and fats. In addition, it has minerals such as calcium and iron, and vitamins such as thiamine and riboflavin. Chocolate becomes even more nutritionally sound when nuts, fruits, and milk are added to it.

- Soon after Brillat-Savarin's pronouncement in 1825 of chocolate as a panacea for mental stress, as well as a restorative for the weak and sick, Parisian apothecaries began to sell chocolate concoctions as **medicine** for the sickly, the scrawny, the nervous, and the overweight.

- "Chocolate contains a very large proportion of **nutritive matter** in a small volume. In an expedition to a great distance, where it is imperatively necessary to reduce the weight of the rations, chocolate offers undeniable advantages."

  –M. Soussingault, *Annales de Physique et du Chimie*

- In "Des Substances Alimentaires," M. Payen wrote, "The cocoa bean has in its composition more nitrogen than wheat flour, about 20 times as much fatty matter, a considerable proportion of starch, and an agreeable aroma which excites the appetite. We are entirely disposed to admit that this substance contains a remarkable **nutritive power**."

- "Chocolate is a **perfect food,** as wholesome as it is delicious, a beneficent restorer of exhausted power; but its quality must be good, and it must be carefully prepared. It is highly nourishing and easily digested, and is fitted to repair wasted strength, preserve health, and prolong life. It agrees with dry temperaments and convalescents; with mothers who nurse their children; with those whose occupations oblige them to undergo severe mental strains; with public speakers, and with all those who give to work a portion of the time needed for sleep. It soothes both stomach and brain, and for this reason, as well as for others, it is the best friend of those engaged in literary pursuits."

—Baron Justus von Liebig (1803-1873),
German chemist and dietetic expert

- Although chocolate is not an aphrodisiac, as the ancient Aztecs believed, chocolate contains **phenylethylamine (PEA)**, a natural substance that is reputed to stimulate the same reaction in the body as falling in love. Hence, heartbreak and loneliness are great excuses for chocolate gorging.

- A treatise on "The Natural History of Chocolate, Being a Distinct and Particular Account of the Cacao Tree, Its Growth and Culture, and the Preparation, Excellent Properties, and Medicinal Virtues of Its Fruits" was written by a French officer who served in the West Indies. It was translated and published in London in 1730. Arguing the value of chocolate in **prolonging life**, he cited this example: "There lately died at Martinico a counselor, about a hundred years old, who for thirty years past lived on nothing but chocolate and biscuit. He sometimes, indeed, had a little soup at dinner, but never any fish, flesh, or other victuals. He was, nevertheless, so vigorous and nimble that at fourscore and five he could get on horseback without stirrups."

- According to U.S. Department of Agriculture statistics, one plain milk chocolate candy bar has more **protein** than a banana, an apple, an orange, a carrot, or a package of seedless raisins.

- "Chocolate in itself is a **pure**, natural food. A finished chocolate product usually has milk and other wholesome ingredients adding to its nutritional content. When items such as peanuts and almonds are incorporated, chocolate's nutritional value is boosted further."

—Patricia Cobe, *Chocolatier* (Vol 1, #1, 1984)

- From its earliest days, chocolate was primarily a beverage, and to it were attributed, according to Susan Heller Anderson (*The New York Times*, December 17, 1980), "many **qualities**: indeed, it was considered an aphrodisiac, a digestive, a soporific, a tonic, even a cure for certain intestinal afflictions."

- A typical 1.5-oz milk chocolate bar contains the following amounts of **Recommended Daily Allowance (RDA)** for just 220 calories:

Nutrient	%RDA
calcium	9
iron	3
protein	6
riboflavin	9
thiamine	1.9
vitamin A	2.4

- Etienne Francois Geoffroy, a distinguished physician and professor of Medicine and Pharmacy in the College of France, wrote in "Traite de Matiere Medicale": "The drinking of chocolate, especially of that made with milk, is **recommended** to persons affected with phthisis or consumption; and, in fact, it supplies a juice which is nourishing, substantial, and smooth, which deadens the acrimony of the humors; provided, as we have said, that the cocoa is properly roasted, and mixed with a very small quantity of spices."

- Edward Bancroft recorded several medical uses for chocolate in his book *Native Races of the Pacific States*. Sometimes, he noted, they were related to **religious ritual**. At other times, the cure was more direct: "Cacao, after the oil had been extracted, was considered to be a sure preventive against poison." (Kolpas, 1978, p. 108).

- Dr. Joseph H. Fries, in "Chocolate: A **Review of Published Reports** of Allergic and Other Deleterious Effects, Real or Presumed" (*Annals of Allergy*, Vol 41, #4, Oct 1978), tried to separate truth from myth: "Chocolate itself can indeed be the incitant in allergic, toxic, and pharmacologic reactions. On the other hand, chocolate would appear to be an easy choice or victim when diagnosis is difficult or obscure and it is blamed and banned promiscuously, often with little justification."

- Chocolate itself is **salt-free** and cholesterol-free.

- Marathon runner **Frank Shorter** reportedly eats a dozen chocolate bars for breakfast and eats several more for extra carbohydrates on days that he is going on long-distance runs.

- "Chocolate, apart from its palatability, has a considerable **stimulating effect** on the heart and the general musculature of the body. It is more than a delicacy; it is good solid food and nourishment and considered as such by many nations. Chocolate is a standard part of army rations in time of stress. Mountaineers carry chocolate with them as a matter of course. French children eat it instead of butter or jam with their bread. And the comfort derived from a chocolate bar when one is tired or depressed is not to be underestimated. It is little wonder that chocolate is America's favorite flavor. Housewives, confronted with a choice of desserts, should remember and when in doubt, make it chocolate."

  –Woman's Day Encyclopedia of Cookery (Fawcett, 1965)

- American and Russian **space flights** have always included chocolate–both for nutritional and morale purposes.

- Lauding chocolate over coffee and tea, Jean Baptiste Alphonse Chevalier wrote: "Cocoa and chocolate are a complete food, coffee and tea are not food. Cocoa gives one third of its weight in starch and one half in cocoa butter; and, converted into chocolate by the addition of sugar, it realizes the idea of a complete aliment, wholesome and eminently hygienic. The shells of the bean contain the same principles as the kernels, and the extract, obtained by an infusion of the shells in sweetened milk, forms a mixture at once agreeable to the taste and an advantageous **substitute for tea and coffee**."

- In addition to chocolate's good qualities for easy digestion, it also has external value for the body in the form of cocoa butter as a **sunbathing cream**. While it won't guard against sunburn, it does help prevent dryness from exposure to the sun.

- *Stedman's Medical Dictionary,* 23rd edition (Williams and Wilkins, 1976) offers these definitions: "**Theobromine**–an alkaloid resembling caffeine in its action, prepared from the dried ripe seed of theobroma cacao or made synthetically; used as a diuretic, myocardial stimulant, dilator of coronary arteries, and smooth muscle relaxant. **Theobroma**–cocoa butter, the fat obtained from the wasted seed of theobroma cacao. It is used as a base for suppositories and ointments, and in operative dentistry, as a lubricant and protective."

- "Using Chocolate in **Therapeutic Diets**," a brochure produced for the Chocolate Manufacturers of the USA, discusses weight control and diabetic, modified fat, renal, and low-sodium diets. A few appropriate recipes are included.

- "I have personal knowledge of 2 or 3 **typhoid fever** patients in hospitals in Cleveland, within the past few weeks, who have been allowed the use of Dutch cocoa 4 to 6 times a day, and have recuperated rapidly on this diet. Cocoa nourishes and builds up the brain and muscle and may be safely used by any member of the family."

  –B. P. Forbes, Forbes Chocolate Company, 1903

- According to Brillat-Savarin, "Chocolate, carefully prepared, is an article of food as **wholesome** as it is agreeable; that it is nourishing, easy of digestion, and does not possess those qualities injurious to beauty with which coffee has been reproached; that it is excellently adapted to persons who are obliged to a great concentration of intellect in the toils of the pulpit or the bar, and especially to travelers; that it suits the most feeble stomach; that excellent effects have been produced by it in chronic complaints, and that it is a last resource in affections of the pylorus."

- About a dozen years ago a concern arose about **xanthine** alkaloids in chocolate, coffee, tea, and cola drinks and their possible effects on benign breast disease. Yet the early studies were criticized for inadequate controls, and later ones have shown that comparisons of before-after mammograms offered little support for a correlation.

- An anonymous traveler from Alaska wrote the following letter to the Walter Baker Company: "While on the toughest mountain trail one of my partners and myself ate nothing from breakfast till supper but your chocolate. We ate about one ounce at a time and finished the day in better shape than those who ate the usual hearty lunch. This might not be generally believed, but members of the **Yukon travellers** can testify to the sustaining powers of cocoa and chocolate."

    –"Cocoa and Chocolate Exhibits," 1915

CHOCOLATE MOGULS

- This comment appeared in a feature article on chocolate in the February 1982 issue of *Town & Country*: "From megaconglomerates to men-with-a-mission–that is the chocolate maker today."

- **American Entrepreneurs Association** of Los Angeles, a business research and development organization, publishes an instruction manual on setting up and operating your own chocolate and/or chocolate cookies shop.

- Founder of **Famous Amos** Chocolate Chip Company, theatrical agent Wally Amos, tells all about it in *The Famous Amos Story: The Face That Launched a Thousand Chips* (Doubleday, 1983). With financial backing from Helen Reddy, Bill Cosby, and Marvin Gaye, Famous Amos went after a small market niche with his premium-priced cookies, sold in gift and specialty food shops. One of the first chocolate chip cookie entrepreneurs, he has become a millionaire in the process.

- Ruth Hanly Booe began making candies with her friend Rebecca Gooch in 1919 as a lark. During prohibition, a friend who managed the Old Frankfort Hotel offered the Kentuckian ladies use of his barroom so they could concoct their confections. Travelers and townspeople alike loved them; **Rebecca-Ruth Candies** was born. A series of setbacks was offset by unique promotion schemes. Ruth bought out her partner in 1929 and ran the business until she turned it over to her son; she died in 1973 at the age of 82. Her son recently announced that a third generation will "carry on the same personal service, satisfaction and quality to each customer that his grandmother always insisted upon so many years ago."

- When he was only 23 years old, **John Cadbury** began his coffee, tea, and cocoa bean business; the year was 1824. Later his brother joined him, then his sons, who introduced the process of Cocoa Essence in 1866. Through a series of mergers and innovations, Cadbury Ltd. today is the world's largest producer of chocolate.

- **Caesar Gabriel Choiseul,** duc de Praslin (1598-1675) was the inventor of the praline. Serving as Secretary of the Navy under Louis XV of France, he was privy to concessions his daughter received from the island of Tortuga. Using ingredients indigenous to the island–chocolate, nuts, brown sugar, vanilla, and tawny rum–Choiseul made a caramel topping for the nuts, then rolled them in chocolate.

- A computer consultant in San Diego, **Frank Crail** decided in 1981 to relocate his family to Durango, Colorado, for a more relaxed lifestyle. Deciding to open a little candy store there, he talked three of his friends into becoming partners and hired a retired candymaker to share his expertise. The result: Rocky Mountain Chocolate Factory. Crail realized the key to success was location: the mystique of chocolate made in the southwest, in a tourist area, near traffic (it is one block from the historic Durango-to-Silverton Railway Station), and a good labor force, and with an open-shop window to demonstrate fudge-making to prospective customers. Sales the first year were $180,000, so three other shops were opened. Within four years Rocky Mountain Candy Factory was a $10 million business, with 10 company-owned stores, 25 franchises, and projections for opening 30 new stores.

- In 1979 David Liederman invested $35,000 to open a cookie shop in Manhattan; within five years, **David's Cookies** had become a $26 million empire, with over 150 franchises in the United States, Japan, Canada, Australia, and England. His secret: chunks of bittersweet chocolate imported from Swiss chocolatier Lindt and Sprungli, plus his notion that "People should be able to smell a cookie, want a cookie, see a cookie, buy a cookie." David's particular marketing strategy is based on entrepreneurial franchising and licensing.

- Debbie Fields, President of **Mrs. Fields** Chocolate Chippery, insists on company-owned-and-operated stores, and has a cookie enterprise based on "feel-good feelings." She started with a single store in Palo Alto, California, in 1977 with $50,000 that she borrowed from her husband. Sales from her more than 500 stores in the United States, Canada, Hong Kong, Japan, Australia, and England add up to $125+ million.

- Wanting to establish a line of kosher chocolate lollipops, **Phillip Gelman** ended up developing the Kosher Chocolate Factory in Northfield, Illinois. In less than a year, he had $250,000 in sales throughout the United States and as far away as South Africa.

- **Domingo Ghiardelli** of Italy began making his chocolates in San Francisco in 1849, and is credited for his patent on the process for making powdered chocolate. His original factory is now the focal point of Ghiardelli Square, a posh collection of elegant shops along Fisherman's Wharf.

- Michael and Susan **Goldman** decided they wanted to do their part for Cultural Survival, a Cambridge, Massachusetts, human rights organization active in the Brazilian rain forest, so they started Toucan Chocolates in 1990. Blending their commitment to the environment and their love of fine chocolates, they decided to "meld the tastes and textures of tropical nuts with the world's best chocolates (light and dark) to create": cashew-caramel tortoises, nut-chocolate clusters, sachew bark, Brazil and cashew nut buttercrunches, and nut caramels. The company, located at 31 Wyman Street in Waban, Massachusetts 02168 (617/964-8696), has already won lots of notice and praise.

- Arriving in California at the time of the Gold Rush, **Etienne Guittard** came to mine but ended up making his fortune from chocolate-making skills he brought with him from his uncle's chocolate factory in Paris. He founded Guittard Chocolate in 1868, and ran it for 31 years. The company has been family-owned and operated ever since.

- When **L. S. Heath** began his confectionery and ice cream business in 1914 in Robinson, Illinois, home freezers had not yet become popular and sales were slow. A pint of hand-dipped ice cream sold for 15 cents. Meanwhile, his sons experimented on the candy-making aspect of the dairy business, and in 1928 developed their formula for "English Toffee." The company today has four of Heath's grandsons actively involved in the organization, and two of his daughters are on the Board of Directors.

- **Milton S. Hershey** (1875-1945) represents the ultimate "pluck and toil" hero of the chocolate industry. In 1876, at the age of 19, he set up a confectionery shop in Philadelphia with $150 borrowed from his Aunt Mattie. Hershey married in 1898, and found himself a millionaire by 1900. He never had any children of his own, but established the Milton Hershey School for unfortunate boys (who had lost one or both parents) in 1909 and the Cuban Orphan School in 1919. When he died at the age of 85, the following eulogy was delivered by Reverend John H. Treder at his funeral: "The life of Milton Hershey will always be an inspiration in the final triumph of records of perseverance, determination, and pure hard work over failure."

- When **Laura Katteman** was ready to graduate as an economics major from college she wanted to start her own business in a major city. Her decision to found the Boston Brownie Company was a fun and profitable one; within five years it was netting $350,000. Located in Boston's Faneuil Hall Marketplace, Boston Brownie offers 25 varieties that retail for $5.95/lb. "Laura's Special" is still the best seller: three layers of fudge buttercream, topped with melted chocolate chips.

- **Rodolph Lindt's** (1855-1909) chocolate factory in Berne, Switzerland, was powered by a water wheel. His genius for invention led him to a process for producing the first melting, or fondant, chocolate. Lindt's other contributions to chocolate history include the refining process known as "conching" and the addition of cocoa butter to chocolate so that it would have the necessary melting quality. When Lindt died, he was still a bachelor, with no children.

- Octogenarian **Forest Mars**, founder of Mars, Inc. wasn't content with having the best-selling candy bar in the United States– Snickers. He recently decided to produce an exquisite "adult" candy bar, filled with liquor, which he produces in Nevada. "Ethyl M" is named for his mother.

- John Mavrakos immigrated to St. Louis in 1907 from Greece and founded **Mavrakos Candies**. Today the company operates more than a dozen stores.

- **Mrs. J. G. McDonald's** Chocolate Company in Salt Lake City, Utah, has been a four-generation family business since 1862. An early entrepreneur, Mrs. McDonald entered several of her candies in world competition, winning 13 ribbons and 44 gold medals over the years.

- Known as "The Truffle Lady," **Alice Medrich** began her Berkeley, California-based company Cocolat in 1976, and has since established an international reputation for herself. There are seven Cocolat shops currently in the Bay Area, employing about 80 people, with more plans for expansion in the works. In 1990, Alice Medrich published a cookbook named for her business, and its top-quality ingredients, unusual recipes, and creative style made it an award-winning success.

- A recent *Ms. Magazine* article featured 17-year-old **Kim Merritt** of Kim's Khocolate Korner in Cumberland, Maryland. What began as a hobby when Kim was eleven has become an 18,000-candy-bars-per-year, $9,000 enterprise. Besides introducing chocolates in every color, Kim handicrafts caramels, pecan turtles, chocolate lace, fudge, and chocolate chip cookies; peanut butter truffles are her most popular product. Besides stylized stationery, Kim's Khocolate Korner also has business cards, stickers, and a professional press kit.

- **Henri Nestle** (1814-1890) of Switzerland invented a milk process for chocolate over a century ago, and right away put his name and trademark–"Little Nest"–on the discovery. His specialty from the start was marketing. Nestle invented the manufacture of children's groats and was the first person to manufacture condensed milk chocolate. The Nestle Company today is the world's largest food corporation.

- When **Frederick Neuhaus** and his wife opened their little candy shop in Brussels in 1851, it quickly became the rage. According to the company, the original ingredients were first-choice cocoa beans, Belgian beet sugar, milk, butter, natural liquor extracts, whole nuts, fruits, and no artificial preservatives whatsoever. The chocolates were considered "miniature works of art." Frederick's grandson, Jean Neuhaus, was the first to develop chocolate praline.

- **Edmond Opler, Sr.**, founder of World's Finest Chocolates, Inc. of Chicago, began his involvement with chocolate at the turn of the century, delivering Runkel's Cocoa by horse and wagon. In 1922 he began his own company, featuring bulk packages of "Our Mother's Cocoa." By 1940, Opler had established World's Finest Chocolate, which specializes in chocolate as a fund-raiser. He also had the foresight to purchase land on the island of St. Lucia, where World's Finest grows its own cocoa and helps support the local farmers. On a videotape recently released by the company, Opler, a nonagenerian is featured praising chocolate as the favorite flavor in the nation and the world; he also commends World's Finest and the people making, selling, and buying it. His son, Ed Opler, Jr., is currently President of the firm.

- Alec Leaver, author of *Making Chocolates* (Weathervane, 1975), comments: "It surely cannot be entirely coincidence that when those gentle and peaceful people, the **Quakers**, were first being persecuted by their fellow Christians, and prevented from entering the professions, a number sought refuge in sweet and chocolate making. So the great names of Rountree, Fry and Cadbury became known throughout the world, not only as chocolate and cocoa manufacturers, but as public benefactors in many fields."

- The year after the Panic of 1893, **Otto J. Schoenleber** of Milwaukee decided to put his local furniture factory, capital, and business experience into the Ambrosia Chocolate Company. With a title that meant "food of the gods" and a favorite axiom of "There is no such word as fail," Schoenleber expanded successfully over the years until his death in 1927 when his daughter, Miss Gretchen B. Schoenleber, became his successor.

- In 1836, **David Sprungli** bought the small pastry shop in Zurich where he was a master confectioner. He and his son Rudolf established a reputation for excellent cakes and confections, and by 1845 their chocolate was being enjoyed by large numbers of Swiss citizens. By the time Rudolf Sprungli retired in 1892, the company's quality chocolate was widely respected. In 1899 Sprungli AG purchased the Lindt Chocolate factory for 1.5 million gold francs; today, the Lindt and Sprungli Chocolate works is run by a sixth generation of Sprunglis.

- Nearly a dozen years ago **Ben Strohecker**, who had been Marketing Director at Schrafts Candy Company, founded Harbor Sweets. With the express purpose of producing "the best piece of candy in the world," Strohecker set out to do market research by asking people, "If you were going to die in the next 10 minutes, what is the last piece of candy you would choose to eat?" The overwhelming answer: chocolate-dipped toffee crunch, followed by chocolate mints, then chocolate-caramel-pecan clusters. Harbor Sweets of Marblehead, Massachusetts, was born. A dozen years later, it is a multimillion-dollar business.

- **Philipp Sucard**, founder of Sucard of Switzerland, studied American candy-making technology in 1824, then returned home to build the first mixing apparatus for chocolate, driven by water power. The Sucard operation today is completely computerized.

- The Union of Swiss Chocolate Manufacturers lists the following as **Swiss chocolate pioneers**: Francois-Louis Cailler, Philipp Suchard, Jacques Foulquier, Charles-Amedee Kohler, Rodolphe Sprungli-Ammann, Aquilino Maestrani, Jacques Klaus, Daniel Peter, Henri Nestle, Johann Georg Munz, Rodolphe Lindt, Alexis Sechaud, Charles Muller and Karl Bernhardt, Jean Tobler, Wilhelm Kaiser, Max Felchlin, and others.

- **Johann Jakob Tobler** began his confectionery apprenticeship in St. Gallen, Switzerland, at the age of 14; by 1867, he had established his own business, in Berne. On the event of his 70th birthday, Jean Tobler turned Tobler Chocolates over to his three children, and it went from a partnership to a joint-stock company in 1902. A subsidiary of Jacobs Suchard AG in Zurich, the company now is a multibillion-dollar coffee and chocolate empire.

- **Casparus J. Van Houten** of the Netherlands was the first person to request a patent for chocolate. Removing about two-thirds of the cocoa butter, he was able to concoct a partially defatted cocoa powder that mixed well with water; the cocoa press was invented. A chemist by background, Van Houten also added potash to his nineteenth century product, a process which alkalized the chocolate powder, making it darker in color, milder in flavor, and more digestible. "Dutch cocoa" is based on Van Houten's discovery.

- The "Whitman Sampler" evolved from **Stephen F. Whitman's** practice of keeping fruits, nuts, and spices available so that customers could specify individualized assortments from his Philadelphia waterfront store in the 1840s. Later, when he moved downtown to serve the Main Line carriage trade, the tradition was maintained. Whitman kept a customer index file so his clientele could "sample" his many chocolate wares, and the famous sampler was developed in 1912. The company has been a division of Pet, Inc. since 1963.

CHOCOLATE QUOTES

- "Everyone seems to have a never-ending **appetite** for chocolate . . . Culinary fads come and go, but chocolate remains . . .

Americans are always going through tidal waves of enthusiasm about food ... Some of these waves crest and then recede, while others seem to get higher and higher. In this latter category, we would certainly place chocolate, the flavor that beats all others.

–Craig Claiborne and Pierre Franey, "Chocolate Mania," *New York Times Magazine*, 1984.

- "Chocolate is a veritable **balm of the mouth**, for the maintaining of all glands and humors in a good state of health. Thus it is, that all who do drink it possess a sweet breath."

–Dr. Stephani Blancardi of Amsterdam, 1705

- "Chocolate makes everybody smile–even **bankers**."

–Ben Strohecker, founder of Harbor Sweets

- "Chocolate truffles are the **black gold** of candydom."

–Jane Salzfass Freiman, writer

- "**Cacaoaquauitl**: This cacao, when much is drunk, when much is consumed, especially that which is green, which is tender, makes one drunk, takes effect on one, makes one dizzy, confuses one, makes one sick, deranges one. When an ordinary amount is drunk, it gladdens one, refreshes one, consoles one, invigorates one. Thus it is said, 'I take cacao. I wet my lips. I refresh myself.'"

–Bernardino de Sahagun, Historia General de las Cosas de Nueva Espana, sixteenth century

- "**Canadians** are chocolate chip all the way."

–Note from "Two Americans to the Canadian Consulate General" in thanks for their help in getting American hostages out of Tehran in 1978.

- "**Caramels** are only a fad. Chocolate is a permanent thing."

–Milton Snavely Hershey

- "What use are **cartridges** in battle? I always carry chocolate instead."

  –The Chocolate Cream Soldier in George Bernard Shaw's
  Arms and the Man (1894)

- "Chocolate is an excellent flavor for ice cream but both unreasonable and disconcerting in **chewing gum**."

  –Fran Leibowitz, *Metropolitan Life* (p. 143)

- "I often dreamed about picking chocolate from a **chocolate tree** and eating my fill."

  –Maida Heatter,
  author of *Book of Great Chocolate Recipes*

- ". . . **communal bites** are the Krazy Glue of life when it comes to keeping good friends together . . . those desserts with names like 'Death by Chocolate' that good friends valiantly help us conquer."

  –Joseph Cohen, American writer

- "Giving chocolate to others is an intimate form of **communication**, a sharing of deep, dark secrets."

  –Milton Zelman, publisher of *Chocolate News*

- ". . . **dark** is to milk chocolate what Don Perignon is to Dr. Pepper."

  –Jenifer Harvey Lang, chef and food writer

- "There's a **difference between chocolate and candy**, and it's important to remember. There's chocolate, which comes solid, like a bar, and then when you take it and wrap it around nuts, sugar, corn syrup, that's candy."

  –Oscar Boldemann, Jr., Boldemann Chocolate Company
  (quoted in Adrianne Marcus, *The Chocolate Bible*,
  G. P. Putnam's, 1979)

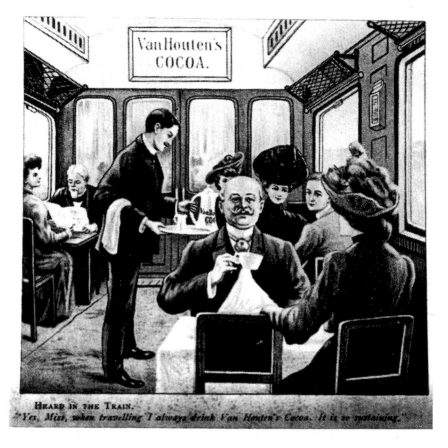

HEARD IN THE TRAIN.
"*Yes, Miss, when travelling I always drink Van Houten's Cocoa. It is so sustaining.*"

- "After a good, complete, and copious breakfast, if we take in addition a cup of well-made chocolate, **digestion** will be perfectly accomplished in three hours, and we may dine whenever we like. Out of zeal for science, and by dint of eloquence, I have induced many ladies to try this experiment. They all declared, in the beginning, that it would kill them; but they have all thriven on it, and have not failed to glorify their teacher."

  –Brillat-Savarin

- "I have completed an analysis of your 'Cocoa Extract,' and find that it is strictly pure, and well manufactured in every way. A portion of the oil has been abstracted, so that your preparation may be easily assimilated by the invalid and as it contains a full-percentage of the vegetable alkaloid with all the other component parts without any admixtures, you can, without any hesitation, recommend your 'Cocoa Extract' for all **domestic and dietetic** purposes."

–W. W. Stoddary, City and County Analyst,
in testimony to J. S. Fry and Sons, 1880

- "Chocolate is my **downfall**."

–Hermione Gingold, actress

- "I am a longtime confirmed chocoholic–I would eat nothing else if I could. My fantasy, I'm afraid, is not terribly wild and outlandish but I **dream** of it constantly: *Krön delivers a 4-pound box of their dark-chocolate truffles and dark-chocolate-covered orange slices every day. The Four Seasons drops off one of their dark-chocolate mousse cakes twice a week. Fresh chocolate-filled croissants, David's Cookies (still warm), and slices of Princess Cake and Opera Cake from Eclair Bakery find their way to my doorstep every morning. Thick, rich chocolate milkshakes miraculously appear in my freezer along with chocolate-mint Girl Scout cookies. And the very best, and most important thing is that I never gain* one ounce *from any of them. Every pound of chocolate I eat makes me look as though I'd spent an hour at the gym! The more you eat, the more fit and slender you become!"*

–Sydney Biddle Barrows ("The Mayflower Madam")

- "Liquidum non frangit jejunum." ([chocolate] liquids, amongst them, do not constitute a break in **fasting**.)

–Cardinal Francis Maria Brancaccio of the Vatican, 1662

- "I just have passed my 85th birthday, and I'm glad I'm not too old to enlist in the cause of the United States. Uncle Sam presented me with the finest present a man could have, the Army

Navy E. The pennant was awarded for producing **Field Ration D**, an emergency ration for our fighters all over the world, developed in collaboration between the U.S. Quartermaster's Department and our laboratories. The patent has been turned over to the U.S. Government. It was just our way of doing what we knew best how to do."

–Milton Snavely Hershey, "There's No Age Limit,"
Everybody's Weekly (October 4, 1942)

- "Few things we eat have as outspoken a **flavor** as chocolate, yet when it is used as a seasoning–as it often is in cuisines other than our own–its character is subdued and one often has a hard time identifying what the subtle flavor is that the chocolate imparts to a dish."

–Michael Field, *All Manner of Food* (Knopf, 1970)

- "I used to DRINK a great deal of chocolate when I was younger. It was about 1924 when I lived in Paris. We had the most BEAUTIFUL chocolate in the morning, with fresh croissants and sometimes those small buns with chocolate in them–au chocolat. Oh, how the French children do love those. Now THAT'S wonderful. HOT CHOCOLATE and THOSE things. What a perfect way to begin a **French day**."

–James Beard,
Chocolatier's premier issue, 1984

- "For who could hate or bear a grudge
Against a luscious bit of **fudge?**"

–Roald Dahl

- "Don't wreck a sublime chocolate experience by feeling **guilty**. Chocolate isn't like premarital sex. It will not make you pregnant. And it always feels good."

–Lora Brody, author of *Growing Up on the Chocolate Diet*

- "The persons who habitually take chocolate are those who enjoy the most equitable and constant **health** and are least liable to a multitude of illnesses which spoil the enjoyment of life."

  –A. Brillat-Savarin, *Physiologie de Gout*

- Describing his ascent of the Lumpa peaks in the **Himalayas**, the highest point ever recorded by man, Henry Savage Landor (1865-1924) wrote: "I had been consuming during the ascent a great many lozenges of highly concentrated meat–each one was supposed to be as good as a meal–and I ate at least 50 in the space of eight hours and a half. I suppose they were sustaining, but one had to eat a great many of them, or they left an awful feeling of emptiness. I had started with my pockets full of Chocolate and what the lozenges could not do the huge chunks of Chocolate I chewed all the way up the mountain certainly accomplished."

- "**Hot fudge** fills deep needs."

  –Susan Isaacs, novelist

- "Always serve too much **hot fudge sauce** on hot fudge sundaes. It makes people overjoyed, and puts them in your debt."

  –Judith Olney, author of *Joy of Chocolate* (Barron, 1982)

- "*Las cosas claras y el chocolate espeso.*" ("**Ideas** should be clear and chocolate thick.")

  –Spanish proverb

- In 1712, Joseph Addison, social satirist of the *Spectator*, warned: "I shall also advise my fair readers to be in a particular manner careful how they meddle with romances, chocolate, novels, and the like **inflamers**, which I look upon as very dangerous to be made use of . . ."

- "America looks upon chocolate as a bonbon. France has always regarded it as a **jewel**."

  –Christian Constant, French chocolatier

- "Take a hundred cacao kernels, two heads of chili or long peppers, a handful of anise or orjevala, and two of mesa chusit or vanilla–or, instead, six Alexandria roses, powdered,–two drachms of cinnamon, and a dozen almonds, and as many hazel-nuts, a half pound of white sugar, and annotto enough to color it, and you have the **king of chocolates**.

–Antonio Colmenero de Ledesma's recipe
for chocolate, 1644

- "What you see before you, my friend, is the result of a **lifetime** of chocolate. A pound a day often."

–Katharine Hepburn

- "The chief use of this cocoa is in a drincke which they call chocolate, whereof they make great account, foolishly and without reason; for it is **loathsome** to such as are not acquainted with it, having a skumme or frothe that is very unpleasant to taste, if they be not well conceited thereof."

–Joseph Acosta, *Historie of the East
and West Indies*, 1604

- "Oh, wouldn't it be **loverly** . . . (to have) lots of choc'late . . . someone's 'ead resting on my knee,/Warm and tender as 'e can be . . ."

–*My Fair Lady*'s Eliza Doolittle

- "I was brought up to believe that you *never* ate chocolate until after **lunch**, and even now am truly shocked at those of my friends who will eat chocolate cake for breakfast, and one who has been known to demolish half a box of the best chocolates before she even gets out of bed in the morning."

–Helge Rubinstein, author of *The Ultimate Chocolate Cake
and 110 Other Chocolate Confections*

- "(William) **McKinley** has no more backbone than a chocolate eclair."

  > –Theodore Roosevelt, in H. T. Peck's *Twenty Years of the Republic*, 1906

- An early Mexican writer discussed the use of cocoa as a **means of exchange**: "It is the best merchandise that is in all the Indies. The Indians make drink of it, and in like manner meat to eat. It goeth currently for money in any market, or fair, and may buy flesh, fish, bread or cheese, or other things."

- "Chocolate is the only food to **melt** exactly at the temperature of the human mouth."

  > –Robert Lambert, cookbook writer and food artist

- "I should have a **musette** full of chocolate. These I should distribute with a kind word and a pat on the back."

  > –Ernest Hemingway

- Alexander Pope's "Rape of the Lock" (1714) alludes to chocolate when he refers to the **negligent spirit**, fixed like Ixion:

  > In fumes of burning chocolate shall glow,
  > And tremble at the sea that froths below.

- In his discussion of various **New World** products, seventeenth century author Arnoldus Montanus describes the value of cocoa: "But much more beneficial is the Cacao, with which Fruit New Spain drives a great Trade; nay, serves for Coin'd Money."

  > –"America: Being the Latest, and Most Accurate Description of the New World," 1671

- "My chocolate fantasy would be that I could eat all the chocolate in every conceivable form that I could possibly ever want and it wouldn't do anything bad to my body or my skin or my disposition. Actually it would have **no calories** at all."

  > –Helen Gurley Brown (*Cosmopolitan*), in Honey and Larry Zisman, *Chocolate Fantasies*, 1988

- **"No other** shall I have."

> –motto for Chocolaterie Corne Toison d'Or

- "I *am* a chocoholic and, as it happens, I do have a favorite chocolate fantasy. It is this–*I would like to be presented with a beautiful red-headed young woman in the **nude** who is covered with a thick layer of bittersweet chocolate. I then remove the chocolate as any red-blooded chocoholic male would.* Not practical, I admit, but a nice fantasy."

> –Isaac Asimov, in Honey and Larry Zisman,
> *Chocolate Fantasies*, 1988

- American pioneer James Wadsworth (1768-1844) wrote the following in *A Curious History of the Nature and Quality of Chocolate*:

> 'Twill make **Old Women** Young and Fresh;
> Create New Motions of the Flesh.
> And cause them long for you know what,
> If they but taste of chocolate.

- "Chocolate is a **perfect** food, as wholesome as it is delicious, a beneficent restorer of exhausted power; but its quality must be good, and it must be carefully prepared. It is highly nourishing and easily digested, and is fitted to repair wasted strength, preserve health, and prolong life. It agrees with dry temperaments and convalescents; with mothers who nurse their children; with those whose occupations oblige them to undergo severe mental strains; with public speakers, and with all those who give to work a portion of the time needed for sleep. It soothes both stomach and brain, and for this reason, as well as for others, it is the best friend of those engaged in literary pursuits."

> –Baron Justus von Liebig (1803-1873),
> German chemist and dietetic expert

- "The improvement of the quality of chocolate was the aim of a French gallant until his unfortunately premature decease. A lady of noble birth, whose honour he was said to have gravely sullied, served him with a cup of **poisoned chocolate**. The suitor calmly emptied the cup, but found time, just before he fell in convulsions, for a technical comment: 'The chocolate would have been better,' he said, 'if you had added a little more sugar; the poison gives it a bitter flavour. Think of this the next time you offer a gentleman chocolate.'"

–Chocosuisse, *Chocologie*, p. 9

- "Chocolate has so many **ramifications**: the politics, the economics, Third World countries' involvement in growing the bean, the psychology of chocolate, the mystique of chocolate, chocolate in music and literature."

–Dr. Herman Berliner, Dean of the School of Business, Hofstra University

- "In a 1903 address to the Cleveland Retail Grocer's Association, B. P. Forbes of the Forbes Chocolate Company made the following statements: "There has been a remarkable increase in the use of cocoa and its products in recent years. Americans consumed nearly $1 million worth of cocoa the last year . . . (and) also consumed over $10 million worth of liquor last year; if these figures could be reversed, making cocoa and chocolate the most popular beverage among our people instead of **rum**, there is no doubt in the speaker's mind that we would see even more rapid scientific progress in the United States, and our laboring classes would be in a better position to enjoy our present prosperity."

- "Any **sane** person loves chocolate."

Bob Greene, newspaper columnist

- ". . . the taste of chocolate is a **sensual** pleasure in itself, existing in the same world as sex . . . For myself, I can enjoy the wicked pleasure of chocolate . . . entirely by myself. Furtiveness makes it better.

"Dr. Ruth" Westheimer

- "Chocolate goes well with **sex**: before, during, after–it doesn't matter."

–Helen Gurley Brown

- "People always say my truffles are better than **sex**."

–Gayle Steinhardt, American chocolatier

- "Chocolate has become very **sophisticated**, not only in quality, but in the way it's packaged. Now people are giving those classic, individual pieces that look like jewels. They're wonderful. Of course, they ought to be at $2.50 a hit!"

–Lora Brody, interview in the *Christian Science Monitor* (2/10/86)

- In his *New Survey of the West Indies* (1648), Thomas Gage describes **Spanish and Indian** ways of making and drinking chocolate: "The cacao and the other ingredients must be beaten in a mortar of stone . . . then with a spoon is taken up some of the paste, which will be almost liquid, and made into tablets, or else without a spoon put into boxes, and when it is cold it will be hard."

- "It is not surprising that **Spanish women** are thin, for there is nothing hotter than the chocolate which they drink to great excess. Furthermore, they season it inordinately with pepper and other spices as much as they are able, so that they do burn themselves."

–Madame d'Aulnoy, 1679

- "**Strength** is the capacity to break a chocolate bar into four pieces with your bare hands–and then eat just one of the pieces."

–Judith Viorst

- "The **superiority** of chocolate drink, both for health and nourishment, will soon give it the same preference over tea and coffee in America which it has in Spain."

  –Thomas Jefferson to John Adams, 1785

- "For who can deny that when the **taste buds** are seeking excitement, drama and sweet satisfaction, it is neither the potato nor the cranberry to which we turn. It is chocolate."

  –Lorna J. Sass, American writer and historian

- ". . . once one is accustomed to chocolate, it is hard to give up drinking it every morning...or in the evening . . . and particularly when one is **travelling**."

  –Francesco Carletti, sixteenth century Florence merchant

- According to Mable Hoffman, author of *Chocolate Cookery* (Dell, 1978), "No other flavor has ever rivaled chocolate in **universal appeal**. Since the days of Montezuma, when the Aztecs drank it from golden goblets in elaborate ceremonies, chocolate has been held in high esteem."

- "**Venice** is like eating an entire box of chocolate liqueurs in one go."

  –Truman Capote

- "Una taza de este precioso brebaje permite un hombre de andar un dia entero sin tomar alimente." ("A cup of this precious beverage permits a man to **walk** an entire day without food.")

  –Cortez, writing to Spain in 1528 about "xocoatl"

- ". . . **watched** chocolate never melts."

  –Pamella Asquith,
  author of *Ultimate Chocolate Cake Book*

CHOCOLATE TIPS

- Most chocolate is best consumed the same day it is purchased–isn't that the **best news** (or excuse!) you've ever heard?!

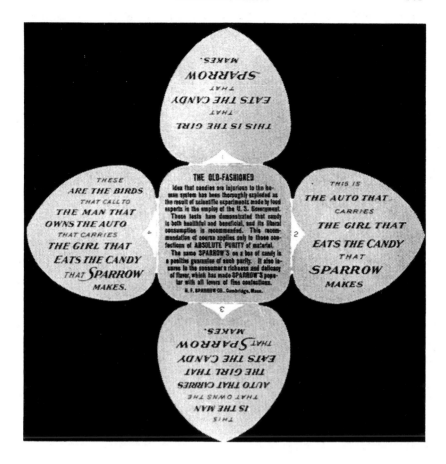

THE OLD-FASHIONED

Idea that candies are injurious to the human system has been thoroughly exploded as the result of scientific experiments made by food experts in the employ of the U. S. Government.

These tests have demonstrated that candy is both healthful and beneficial, and its liberal consumption is recommended. This recommendation of course applies only to those confections of ABSOLUTE PURITY of material.

The name SPARROW'S on a box of candy is a positive guarantee of such purity. It also insures to the consumer's richness and delicacy of flavor, which has made SPARROW'S popular with all lovers of fine confections.

H. F. SPARROW CO., Cambridge, Mass.

THESE ARE THE BIRDS THAT CALL TO THE MAN THAT OWNS THE AUTO THAT CARRIES THE GIRL THAT EATS THE CANDY THAT *SPARROW* MAKES.

THIS IS THE AUTO THAT CARRIES THE GIRL THAT EATS THE CANDY THAT *SPARROW* MAKES

THIS IS THE GIRL THAT EATS THE CANDY THAT *SPARROW* MAKES.

THIS IS THE MAN THAT OWNS THE AUTO THAT CARRIES THE GIRL THAT EATS THE CANDY THAT *SPARROW* MAKES.

- When chocolate becomes too warm during storage, it can develop a whitish film on the surface called "**bloom**," which consists of the finest traces of melted cocoa butter. While bloom doesn't affect baking performance or the flavor of your chocolate, it can mar the appearance of some items.

- **"Candy kinks"**–to obtain a creamy texture, beat all cocoa candy after removing from stove.

–Runkel's Cocoa Cookery, 1870

- Chef Martin Johner offers invaluable technical hints for chocolate decorations, such as the triangular wedges known as **"caravelle"** in his and Gary Goldberg's *Mountains of Chocolate* (Chalmers, 1981).

- For every four ounces of regular baking chocolate, **Julia Child** suggests adding one ounce of bittersweet chocolate.

- To make **chocolate curls:** dip a long, narrow vegetable knife into hot water, then run the knife along the edge of sweet or semi-sweet chocolate.

- Always use a **dry container** for melting chocolate. Try these methods:
  1. double boiler
  2. water bath
  3. microwave oven

- When baking a chocolate cake, instead of **dusting** the greased pan with flour, use cocoa–it looks, and tastes, much better!

- "A box of chocolate confections at hand for nibbling is a joy at any time. A box of chocolate cookies in the freezer takes care of many an **emergency**."

  –Gertrude Parke (A & W Visual Library, 1968)

- Cures for **fear of fudge-making:**
  1. Don't make fudge on a rainy or humid day.
  2. Use a pan that holds four times the volume of the heated ingredients.
  3 Use a good candy thermometer and a wooden spoon.
  4. Score while still warm.
  5. Enjoy!

- According to *Chocologie*, a publication of the Chocolate Industry in Switzerland, the **hallmark** of good chocolate can be detected when you break off a piece: "it breaks firmly and crisply, the edges are clean and the surfaces of the break do not crumble away."

- To **increase the flavor** of chocolate, Brillat-Savarin divulges the secret which Madame d'Arestrel, Mother Superior of the Convent of the Visitation at Belley, revealed to him: "When you want to taste good chocolate," said the religious gourmande, "make it the night before, in a faience coffee pot, and leave it. The chocolate becomes concentrated during the night and this gives it a much better consistency."

- According to **Madame Chocolate** of Chicago, chocolate "can be melted, formed, shaped, curled, grated, drizzled, molded, scraped, coated, frozen, baked, dipped, sprinkled, sculpted."

- Custom confectioner Marge Kehoe says the following **materials** are necessary for a first chocolate session: double boiler, spoon, fork, wax paper, scissors, sandwich bags, chocolate candy wafers–dark, milk chocolate or white, all specially tempered for candymaking–and molds, if desired.

- Quality chocolate **melts in your mouth** like butter, neither clinging to the palate nor feeling gritty on the tongue.

- **Melting chocolate** works best when it is broken or chopped into pieces; it melts more evenly. White chocolate should be well chilled, then finely ground, before melting.

- Since chocolate is highly susceptible to **odors**, it should be carefully wrapped and stored at a distance from foreign flavors. White chocolate is especially prone to taking on new odors, and will turn rancid if exposed to prolonged light.

- Chef Martin Johner of the Culinary Center of New York states that there are two basic **principles** to remember when working with chocolate:

  1. Chocolate burns easily.
  2 Chocolate and water don't always mix.

- **Refrigeration** can sometimes do chocolate more harm than good. Ideally it should be stored at 78°, but at any rate room temperature will rarely turn it rancid.

- *LOVE: Chocolate Recipes* by Kristin Elliott (Beverly, Massachusetts) suggests using a vegetable knife or potato parer on a square of baking chocolate for making **chocolate shavings**.

- Good chocolate should **smell** like chocolate, not cocoa.

- *The Cook's Catalogue* (Harper & Row, 1975) suggests using boxwood and cherrywood **chocolate spoons**, "designed for stirring bubbly hot chocolate in tall porcelain pots"–especially since they don't conduct heat or give off any flavors to the brew.

- Chocolate can be **stored** for a relatively long period of time, provided it is kept in a cool, moisture-free place (about 60°-70° Fahrenheit, 12-18° Centigrade) in the unopened packaging.

- For **substitutions:**

  3 Tablespoons cocoa
       plus   = 1 oz unsweetened baking chocolate
  1 Tablespoon butter

- For each 6 oz cup of **semisweet chocolate pieces,** you can substitute: 2 oz unsweetened chocolate, 7 Tablespoons sugar, and 2 Tablespoons shortening.

- Helmut Loibl, an instructor at the Culinary Institute of America, suggests chopping chocolate and putting it over a double boiler at a low temperature to melt it. To **temper** chocolate, don't let it go above 86°.

- Try not to have too many variations in **temperature** for your chocolate.

- **Tempering**, the process of temperature-controlling the cocoa butter structure of a chocolate mixture, is used for dipping or molding processes. Ideal temperatures of tempering are:

dark chocolate	88°-91°
milk chocolate	84°-87°
white chocolate	84°-87°

- **Timing** of melted chocolate is critical. Sweet chocolate, milk chocolate, and white chocolate should be used immediately; unsweetened and semisweet chocolate can be kept for up to about ten minutes after melting.

- Botanical writer Mel Hunter has written an instructive article on "Growing Your Own **Cocoa Tree**" in the March 1987 issue of *Chocolatier.*

- Joan Lipkis offers "The **Ultimate Chocolate** Candy Classes"– molding, piping, hand-dipping, rolling, and creating with chocolate. Contact her at The King's Chocolate House, 112-09 Rockaway Blvd., Ozone Park, New York 11420, 718/848-8564.

- Unsweetened chocolate can be thickened, if necessary, by carefully adding drops of **vanilla extract**. Stir well.

CHOCOLATE TRIVIA

- In the United States, only three states allow the addition of **alcohol** (up to one-half of one percent) to chocolate: Nevada, Kentucky, and Tennessee. The liquor-filled chocolate can only be purchased in-state, and is not available for mail orders.

- There are more than 2,130 chocolate shops in **Belgium**, a country which has annual per capita consumption of chocolate of 23-24 lbs (as opposed to nearly 10 lbs per person in the United States.) Belgium has an annual chocolate production rate of more than 135,000 tons.

- **Brazil** was the site of the first cocoa plantations. Beginning in 1822, it became a leader in world cocoa markets within a few decades.

- Rebecca-Ruth Candies, founded in 1919 in Frankfort, Kentucky, was the first company to ever produce candy made with 100-proof **bourbon whiskey**.

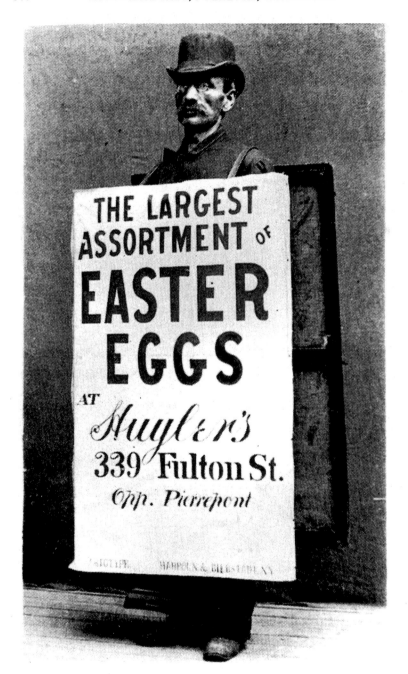

- The **first recipe for brownies** appeared in the 1896 edition of the *Fannie Farmer Cookbook*. The next year, Sears & Roebuck included one in their catalogue.

- The first illustration of the **cacao tree** was described in Girolamo Benzoni's book *The History of the New World*, which was originally published in Venice in 1565. A tropical plant thriving only in hot, rainy climates, the cacao tree is unique in that its flowers and fruits cluster on both its branches and trunk. It is indigenous to Central and South America, plus the west coast of Africa. Each cacao tree pod contains 20 to 40 cacao beans.

- In 1896 **Cadbury** of Birmingham, England, first advertised its "Cocoa Essence"; today a division of Cadbury-Schweppes, Ltd., it is the world's largest producer of chocolate.

- Ray Brockel, author of *The Chocolate Chronicles*, claims that some 70% of the **candy bars** now being produced are chocolate-covered, while many others include chocolate in their ingredients.

- The first **"chocolate box"** was introduced by Richard Cadbury in 1868 when he decorated a candy box with a painting of his young daughter Jessie holding a kitten in her arms. Cadbury also invented the first Valentine's Day candy box.

- At last count, chocolate was determined to contain about **1,200 chemical compounds**. Some 369 volatile compounds have been identified in roasted cocoa beans.

- On July 30, 1502, in Nicaragua, on his fourth trip to the New World, **Christopher Columbus** became the first European to discover cocoa beans–which he brought back to the court of King Ferdinand of Spain.

- The **"conching"**/blending process for premium chocolates can take up to 72 hours a batch, while it only takes about nine minutes to blend assembly-line chocolates.

- Page and Shaw of Boston, in operation since 1888, have as their motto: "Our business methods are an open book to everyone."

They were the first company to use modern refrigerating methods in **dipping chocolate**.

- Chocolate can be deadly for **dogs**. Most dangerous of all is baking chocolate, which contains about 10 times the active ingredient of milk chocolate, theobromine. One ounce of cooking chocolate, even part of a 1-pound bag of candy-coated chocolate, can be life-threatening to a canine weighing up to 10 pounds. The following helpful chart appeared in a February 1991 article in *Better Homes and Gardens*:

Amount of Chocolate That Could be Dangerous to Dogs

Pet	Baking chocolate	Milk chocolate
5 pounds (Yorkshire terrier)	1/2 ounce (1/2 square)	5 ounces (4 avg. candy bars)
10 pounds (miniature poodle)	1 ounce (1 square)	10 ounces (1 jumbo candy bar)
25 pounds (cocker spaniel)	2 1/2 ounces (2 1/2 squares)	25 ounces (2-lb. bag)
50 pounds (dalmatian)	5 ounces (5 squares)	50 ounces (3 pounds)
75 pounds (German shepherd)	7 1/2 ounces (7 1/2 squares)	75 ounces (about 10 jumbo bars)

- **Eichenberger** Confiserie and Tea Room on the Bahnhofplatz in Berne boasts of being the oldest confectionery store in Switzerland.

- **France** was the first country to use mechanical devices to manufacture chocolate, while **Germany** claims that the first place on record to manufacture chocolate was in Steinhude.

- The world's largest producer of raw cocoa beans for commercial use is **Ghana**. Missionaries planted the first cocoa trees there about a century ago, and today they account for more than half the world's crop of cocoa beans.

- When Johann Wolfgang **von Goethe** toured Switzerland in 1797, he brought his own chocolate and chocolate pot.

- The world's first combination bar was Standard Candy Company of Nashville's **Goo Goo Cluster**. A mixture of caramel, marshmallows, peanuts, and milk chocolate, it was developed in 1912.

- **Hebert's Candy Mansion** on Route 20 in Shrewsbury, Massachusetts, established in 1946, was the first roadside candy store in the United States.

- When De Rigeur, a 4-year-old gelding who was a 20-to-1 outsider, won the Balmoral Handicap at Ascot race course in England in 1987, he was disqualified from the $15,000 prize money when the Jockey Club, governing body of British **horseracing**, found he had eaten a Mars bar. A routine urine test after the race turned up traces of theobromine from the chocolate, which contains the stimulant, expressly prohibited under the sport's anti-doping laws. Although a stable girl had given the thoroughbred the sweet, the trainer was fined $860. The only comparable incident in Britain occurred in 1980, when No Bombs was disqualified from a race after snatching a chocolate bar from a stable boy.

- It was **King Louis XIV** of France who first established the position of "Royal Chocolate Maker to the King."

- There is controversy over whether the **first (completely) machine-made chocolate** was produced in Barcelona in 1780 or in Paris by Monsieur Debauve, chocolate maker to the king.

- Currently, chocolate **manufacturers** use 40% of the almonds, 20% of the peanuts, and 8% of the sugar in the world.

- According to the Chocolate Manufacturers of America, its chocolate manufacturers use about 3,500,000 pounds of whole **milk** each day to make milk chocolate.

- **Milk chocolate** accounts for 80% of all the chocolate that Americans consume on a daily basis, or 1.17 billion pounds per year.

- The **first chocolate mill** in the United States was established in 1765, "set upon the bank of the Neponset River at Dorchester, Massachusetts"; it became Walter Baker and Company.

- More than 240 million chocolate **morsels** are purchased every day in the United States.

- Different cultures'/countries' **names** for chocolate:

Americans	chocolate
Armenians	shokolat
Aztecs	chocotyl
French	chocolat
Germans	schokolade
Italians	cioccolata
Mexicans	chocolatl
Portuguese	chocolate
Russians	shokoladno
Spanish	chocolate

- **Napoleon** Bonaparte reputedly always carried chocolate with him during times of battle–for quick energy.

- "The quintessential Belgian chocolate," **Neuhaus** is the world's oldest confectioner still making chocolates by hand; the company began in 1857.

- **Oxford** was the site in 1650 of the first recorded drinking of chocolate in England.

- Traditionally, **Parisians** eat chocolate fish in anticipation of April Fool's Day.

- It takes two pounds of cocoa beans to **produce** one pound of cocoa powder, but only 10 ounces of beans to produce one pound of chocolate.

- Chocolate is the #1 best seller at theatre candy counters; **Raisinettes** are the favorite.

- **Salt Lake City**, Utah, is reputed to have the highest candy consumption per person than any other place in the United States. They love their chocolate!

- In the bar category of confections, M&M/Mars' **Snickers** bar remains the biggest seller, followed by Hershey's Reeses' Peanut Butter Cups.

- When **Chocolat Sprungli** took over the factory of Rodolphe Lindt in 1899, the price paid for its equipment, secret recipes, and trademark rights was 1.5 million gold francs.

- **"Surfin,"** a classic bittersweet chocolate confection, was the world's very first chocolate bar, invented in 1879 by Rodolphe Lindt by means of a "Lindt-conche" machine that eliminated the natural bitterness of the cocoa bean.

- A telephone **survey** conducted in May 1984 among a national probability sample of 1,003 households by Opinion Research Corporation on behalf of the Chocolate Manufacturers Association of America found: "Over 8 in 10 households surveyed contain at least one individual who eats desserts, snacks, or drinks beverages made with or containing chocolate."

- The **Swiss** consume more chocolate per person than any other country in the world. The country's first chocolate factory was built in 1819 in Corsier, near Vevey, by Francois-Louis Cailler. Swiss chocolate makers are legally bound to use their country's own raw materials, many of which are price-controlled.

- The **United States** is the #1 producer of chocolate in the world, followed by West Germany, the Netherlands, and Great Britain. It also leads the world in cocoa bean imports. Pennsylvania produces more chocolate than any other state in the U.S.

- When the **University of California at Berkeley** offered a course on the botanical aspects of cocoa production, more than 800 students signed up for the 35-seat class.

- The Guinness Book of Records reports that the **world's largest chocolate sculpture** was Red Tulip Chocolate's 10+ foot, 4,484-lb chocolate Easter egg constructed in Melbourne, Australia, in 1978. It took two weeks to build.

CHOCOLATE TYPES

- **Bittersweet** chocolate, not to be confused with unsweetened or semisweet chocolate, is primarily used in baking. A slightly sweetened dark chocolate, it has many uses, such as for shiny chocolate curls as garnishes or rich, dense chocolate cakes. Both it and semisweet chocolate are required by law to contain at least 35% chocolate liquor.

- The mashed fruit of a Mediterranean pine tree, **carob** has a flavor that approximates chocolate's flavor. Although not the real thing, carob can be used for people searching for a chocolate substitute.

- **Chocolate sprinkles**, small cylindrical decorating chocolate pieces, are mainly used for cake and cookie decorating, candy, and ice cream cone-dipping.

- **Cocoa** is the result of removing most of the cocoa butter from chocolate liquor by hydraulic pressure. Pure unsweetened cocoa is often used in baking because of its easy blendability with dry ingredients. Some cocoa powder is used pharmaceutically or in the manufacture of beauty aids. "Dutch process" cocoa, which neutralizes the acidity in the powder, makes it more digestible, darker in color, and stronger in flavor. West Africa produces about one-third of the world's cocoa, with the rest coming principally from Brazil, Ecuador, Venezuela, and Malaysia. According to the Coffee, Sugar, and Cocoa Exchange, the leading cocoa importing nations are the United States, West Germany, the Netherlands, the U.S.S.R., and the United Kingdom. Baron Alexander von Humboldt (1769-1859), who conducted scientific journeys in the South American, Cuban, and Mexican hemispheres, proposed the still-accepted theory that cocoa was indigenous to the forests of the Amazon and Orinoco. The cocoa tree belongs to the natural order of "sterculiaceae," a family of about 41 genera and 521 species found inhabiting warmer regions of the world.

- Today, world production of **cocoa beans** is currently estimated at 850,000 tons per year, with Ghana the world leader; Brazil, Nigeria, the Cameroons, the Ivory Coast, the Dominican Republic, Ecuador, Venezuela, Mexico, Columbia, Panama, Guatemala, Costa Rica, Nicaragua, Trinidad, and Haiti are lesser but important producers. Ninety percent of all cocoa beans grown today are classified as "forastero"; only 10% are known as "criollo"

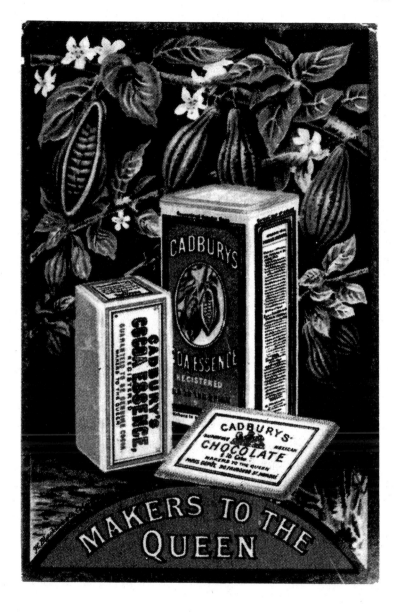

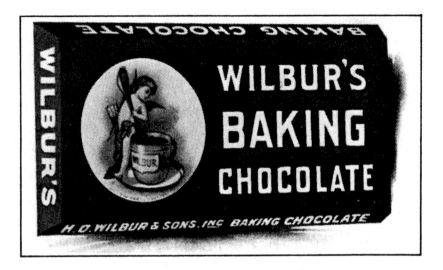

and "arriba," the finer flavor grades. Some of the rarest and most costly cocoa beans are grown in the Lake Maracaibo region of Venezuela.

- **Cocoa butter**, a complex, hard fat made up mostly of triglycerides, remains firm at room temperature, then contracts as it cools and solidifies. It is ideal for molding.

- Early in the eighteenth century, Europeans ate and drank chocolate in different **concoctions**, such as oatmeal chocolate, acorn chocolate, barley chocolate, icelandic-moss chocolate, and rice chocolate.

- **"Couverture,"** is not a brand of chocolate, but rather a term for a coating chocolate used by professional bakers for its shiny, smooth quality. It contains more cocoa butter than regular chocolate. The finest couverture maintains a smooth texture and a well-balanced flavor.

- The Food and Drug Administration (FDA) supplies information on the **"Definition and Standards"** for chocolate and cocoa.

- **Dietetic chocolate** is sweet, bittersweet, or milk chocolate made with sorbitol or mannitol in place of sugar. Meant for people on sugar-restricted diets and not weight watchers, dietetic chocolate can actually be more caloric than regular chocolate.

- The **Encyclopedia Britannica** defines chocolate this way: "a food product made from cocoa beans that have been fermented, roasted, cracked open, and separated from the shells and germs, leaving the nibs, or kernel fragments, which are ground to form a paste called chocolate liquor. Chocolate liquor may be hardened in molds to form baking (bitter) chocolate; pressed to reduce the cocoa butter (vegetable fat) content and then pulverized to make cocoa powder; or mixed with sugar and additional cocoa butter to make sweet (eating) chocolate developed by the English firm of Fry & Sons in 1847. The addition of concentrated milk to sweet chocolate produces milk chocolate, introduced by Daniel Peter of Switzerland in 1876."

- What separates good chocolate from the average is determined by the amount of cocoa butter added. The **finest chocolate** starts with the beans, and the best beans come from South America, primarily Ecuador.

- Chocolate **fudge** topping, a mixture of cocoa, sugar, corn syrup, and flavorings with milk, cream, and/or butter, is usually (fantastically!) heated and poured over ice cream.

- Swiss **"ganache"** is their invention that is made from a combination of the very freshest possible cream and finest-quality chocolate.

- **German chocolate** is a special blend of chocolate with sugar and cocoa butter. Usually available in 4-oz bars grooved into 18 sections, this sweet cooking chocolate is not to be confused with milk chocolate candy.

- Combinations of cocoa, sugar, and milk solids make up **hot cocoa mix**, a fast beverage made by the addition of hot water or milk. It can usually be purchased in individual envelopes, or in bulk, regular, or artificially pre-sweetened forms.

- **Milk chocolate** is sweetened chocolate with dried milk powder and flavorings added. Heavy additions of milk products make

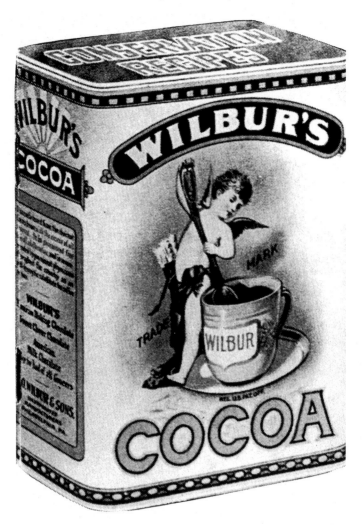

this chocolate more temperamental to work with than semisweet chocolate. Daniel Peter of Switzerland put the first milk chocolate on the market in 1875. Legally, it must contain at least 25% cocoa components and 14% milk, but the sugar content should not exceed 55%. Because it contains a lesser amount of chocolate liquor, milk chocolate cannot be substituted for dark chocolate in recipes calling for bittersweet, sweet, or semisweet chocolate.

- Jewish dietary laws prescribe **"kosher"** foods, which in the case of chocolate can be purchased at, among other places: Kosher Chocolate Factory in Chicago; Sweethearts Three in Chestnut Hill, Massachusetts; Paron Chocolatier in Scarsdale, New York; Karl Bissinger in St. Louis; Wilbur Chocolate Company in Lititz, Pennsylvania; Milton York in Long Beach, Washington; Dilettante in Seattle; and World's Finest Chocolate in Chicago.

- Although creme de cacao is the most popular **chocolate liqueur**, there are also cherry, mint, coconut, and orange-flavored chocolate liqueurs.

- **"Praline,"** a confection made of ground almonds or hazelnuts and sugar for chocolates, is named for the French Duke of Plessis-Praslin, who named the concoction in 1671. Europeans use the term "praline" to mean individual pieces of a variety of fine chocolates.

- **Pre-melted** unsweetened baking chocolate, a blend of cocoa and vegetable oil, is available in one-ounce packets that can be squeezed out and used for baking, with or without melting or measuring.

- A recent chemical breakthrough in chocolate analysis revealed **"pyrazines,"** the stuff that gives chocolate its bitter and nutty taste.

- Ecole Ritz-Escoffier of Paris has offered courses on chocolate, and there are a number of **chocolate schools** in the U.S., like Joan Lipkis' King's Chocolate House in Ozone Park, New York, or *Chocolatier*'s Dessert School.

- Variously known as chocolate bits, chips, or morsels, **semisweet chocolate pieces** are unsweetened chocolate blended with sugar, cocoa butter, and flavorings. They usually come in 6-oz bags, which contain one cup of chocolate pieces, or 12-oz/2-cup bags.

- **Superchocolates** are distinguished from ordinary bonbons by a lengthier conching period, hand-dipping (vs. being sprayed with chocolate), and having no artificial preservatives.

- **Sweetened chocolate** includes bittersweet, semisweet, and sweet chocolates, with sugar added in increasing amounts. These chocolates can also be used in baking but are especially ideal too for decorative piping, molding, spreading, dipping, and, of course, eating. They take the form of squares, chips, or solid candy bars. Bulk sweetened chocolates, called "couvertures," are usually sold in 10-lb slabs.

- Although they have experimented for decades, food scientists have been unable to develop **synthetic chocolate**. It may be an impossibility anyway, since chocolate contains hundreds of different substances, and to date researchers remain baffled at their reproduction.

- Chocolate-flavored **syrup**, a mixture of cocoa, sugar, corn syrup, and flavorings, is used as a sauce, topping, or in beverages.

- Various cultures have altered chocolate to suit their own particular **tastes**. The Aztecs added spices to it, because they liked it with a bitter taste. Spaniards preferred chocolate sweeter, and added sugar. The Italians enjoyed it with liquid, especially hot. It was the English who added milk to chocolate, to be enjoyed as a warm and frothy beverage. Luckily, the Swiss invented milk chocolate for eating.

- **Unsweetened chocolate** is pure chocolate liquor, with no sugar added. Consisting of cocoa powder and cocoa butter, it is also called bitter chocolate or baking chocolate, and is used primarily for baking purposes. According to the U.S. Standard of Identity, unsweetened chocolate is required to consist of a minimum of 50% and a maximum of 58% cocoa butter.

- **White chocolate** is not considered real chocolate, because although it has cocoa butter, it does not have chocolate liquor. In composition, white cocoa butter coating is similar to milk chocolate, since it has extra milk products. The Food and Drug Administration (FDA) has declared it illegal to label food as white chocolate. According to a 1984 policy statement by Taylor Quinn, Associate Director of the FDA, "We have consistently advised that the name 'white chocolate' applied to a product containing no chocolate misbrands the food." Yet, a white chocolate mousse served recently at the trend-setting Palace Restaurant in New York City reportedly has sent interest-waves throughout the industry, and some observers think "mousse apartheid" will become a thing of the past!

Chapter IV

Chocolate Fantasies

CHOCOHOLISM

- "A true chocolate lover finds ways to **accommodate his passion** and make it work with his lifestyle. One key, not just to keeping weight down and staying guilt-free, but also to keeping taste buds sharp (essential for the professionals who evaluate new products as well as judge recipes), is being discriminating."

  –Julie Davis of the *Los Angeles Times*, 10/30/85

- "Although there's no pharmacological evidence that chocolate is **addictive**," writer Judith Stone has commented, "people in thrall to the substance do goofy things."

- According to Honey and Larry Zisman, **Americans** eat this much chocolate:

100	pounds every second
6,000	pounds every minute
360,000	pounds every hour
8,500,000	pounds every day
60,000,000	pounds every week
250,000,000	pounds every month
3,000,000,000	pounds every year

- Focus groups in New York, Chicago, and Los Angeles interviewed by J. K. Fuchs and Associations about their **attitudes toward chocolate** offered these responses:

"Chocolate is fun!"

"Chocolate is one of those 'little extras' I allow myself, even when I can't afford a new suit."

"Chocolate is my passion. I love it."

"Chocolate is sexy. I especially enjoy sharing it with my boyfriend in bed."

"It makes me feel special, and when I give good chocolate as a gift, I can see it makes (the recipient) feel special, too!"

"Chocolate is like 'forbidden fruit.' I know I shouldn't eat it, 'cause of its bad effects, but I can't stay away."

- **"The Chocoholic's Creed"** is included in Madame Chocolate's 5th-edition catalogue: "I admit that I am a chocoholic. I am unable to control the voice within me that says 'truffle' (who wants to fight it anyway?) I promise to endure a never-ending quest for the perfect fudge and will continue to criticize restaurants that do not put chocolate on their menus. I will never criticize a fellow chocoholic who may like it dark though I like milk; and I will always look sideways at a friend who orders vanilla ice cream. Finally, I pledge to hold my head up high when I dunk Oreos into cocoa as I say 'I am a chocoholic and I am proud!' "

- The Swiss Colony of Monroe, Wisconsin, puts out a **"Chocoholic's Survival Kit,"** consisting of: 10 V.I.P. Chocolate Tags, 3 oz of Chocolate Butter Toffee, 1 3/4 oz of V.I.P. Chocolate Assortment, and 2 oz of Chocolate Peanut Clusters.

- A public health nutritionist on a Chocolate Binge Weekend observed, "It's funny, I always wondered what a group of **chocoholics would look like**. They're not particularly heavy–in fact, some are quite lean. They come from all professions. They're friendly and quite intelligent. FINALLY, I'm in a group of kindred spirits who truly UNDERSTAND."

–quoted in the *New York Times* (February 9, 1982)

- Choco-Holics Unanimous of Niles, Illinois, offers **"Choco-Holic™ Relief Spray."**

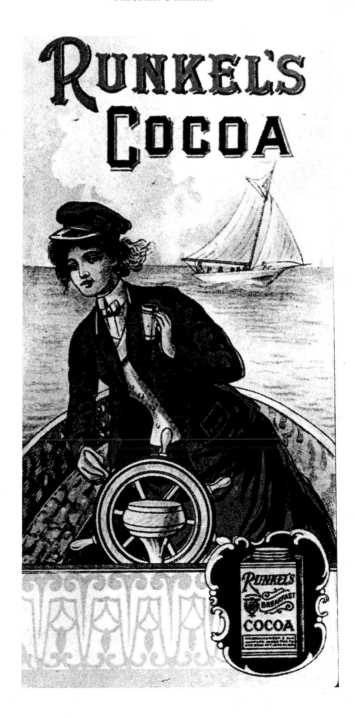

- "People with a high risk of **chocolate addiction** sometimes devise elaborate strategies to keep from becoming hooked, like California chocolatier Mary Vulkanic, who won't eat chocolate on Wednesdays and Fridays. June Mennell, owner of Palm Beach's Fun-in-the-Sun Chocolate Shop, says the trick is 'having enough brains to know when to stop.' She stops when she's had a pound. But many chocolate abusers find that kind of self-discipline beyond them, and can cure themselves only by going, as it were, cold bunny."

  –Newsweek (April 4, 1983), p. 53

- "I love chocolate in any form," says Ray Bolger (*Chocolate News*, May/June, 1982), "from cocoa to chocolate candy, but most of all I love **chocolate cake**, with a rich, creamy mouth-watering chocolate frosting and a chocolate fudgy filling (not too skimpy on the chocolate please.) The cake must be dark, chocolate dark."

- "The chocolate addict of today may raid the Hershey bars at the corner store to satisfy his cravings but some have graduated to being **chocolate connoisseurs** as premium chocolates become more available and well known."

  –Kathy and Clara Li Donni, news correspondents
  for the *Middlesex* (Massachusetts) *News*
  (August 24, 1984)

- "Five years ago, hoping to kick a **chocolate habit** that was significantly affecting my life, I enrolled in a program at the Schick Center for the Control of Smoking, Alcoholism, and Overeating, in Los Angeles. I was then 33. I could not remember the last time I had managed to get through a whole day without eating chocolate in one form or another, usually in quantities most people would regard as excessive, if not appalling . . . Frankly, I am mystified by what happened and to this day cannot explain it. Being addicted to chocolate was so much a part of my definition of myself that it constantly amazes me to think that I am now free of it."

  –38-year-old woman, social worker, in Weil and Rosen,
  From Chocolate to Morphine (Houghton-Mifflin, 1983)

- The introduction to *Beverly Hills Chocolate Recipes*, edited by Barbara Wolf, is a copy of the **Chocolate Lovers' Pledge**: "I would readily give my life for only three things . . . the safety of my family, the protection of my country, and a good piece of chocolate."

- Today **chocolate lovers range** from the affluent seekers of the good life to the kid at the candy corner. The food that chocoholics crave ranges from extravagantly lush (and extravagantly priced) assortments down to simple 'chocolate bars'–which may actually contain no chocolate at all."

  –Gordon Young, *National Geographic* (November 1984)

- You can needlework a **chocolate sampler** featuring a huge Hershey's Kiss in the middle, surrounded by smaller ones, and commanding, "KISS ME . . . I'm a chocoholic."

- Maida Heatter describes her fantasy in her *Book of Great Chocolate Desserts* (Knopf, 1980): "I often dreamed about picking chocolates from a **chocolate tree** and eating my fill."

- Joan Steuer, editor of *Chocolatier* magazine, prefers the term **"chocophile"** to chocoholic, claiming many chocolate lovers don't randomly pop bonbons into their mouths, but consider gourmet items like truffles an indulgence, "not something to stuff your face on."

- Broadway and movie actor **James Coco**, whose very name indicates something of his habit, shares his ultimate chocolate fantasy: "First take a big loaf of Italian bread and slice it in half lengthwise. Then layer in cheese, salami, ham, bologna–and cover the top with chocolate bars."

- Janice Wald Henderson offers a Chocolate Personality Quiz in *Chocolatier* (Vol. 1, #3, 1984) that describes a Type A **Consummate Chocophile:** your chocolate purchases are premeditated, and are usually for bittersweet chocolate–"rich and dark, extra-smooth and outrageously intense . . . You will consume them, and with lavish–almost ritualistic–ceremony . . . You're adamant that chocolate and romance go together . . . You possess strong chocolate preferences . . . Your secret fantasy? To discover that your long-lost uncle is Chairman of the Board of a gourmet chocolate company."

- "The people who make **constant use of chocolate** are the ones who enjoy the most steady health, and are the least subject to a multitude of little ailments which destroy the comfort of life; their plumpness is also more equal."

  –Brillat-Savarin

- "When you **crave chocolate**, you crave chocolate," declares Dana Davenport, owner of Dilettante Chocolates in Seattle (in *Chocolatier*'s premier issue). "Chocolate should be resistive to your bite–not light and fluffy, but dark and rich. The chocolate shell coating should have a snap crunch and slight tooth resistance with each bite."

- Chocolate publisher Milton Zelman admits, "I **dream** about chocolate twenty-four hours a day."

- "Chocolate. Everybody likes it, a lot of people love it, real chocoholics lust after it. And **February 14** wouldn't be the same without it."

  –Gail Perrin of the *Boston Globe* (February 5, 1985)

- **Hermione Gingold** talks about chocolate in *Chocolate News* (March/April, 1981): "I love it. It's my downfall. I absolutely adore it, ever since I was a child up in the nursery. We used to have chocolate scraped on bread and butter."

- At age 70, **Katharine Hepburn** told *Time* magazine, "I don't have to watch my figure as I never had much of one to watch. What you see before you is the result of a lifetime of eating chocolate." Her favorite: dark, pudding-like brownies.

- "I wouldn't dare keep a box (of chocolate) at my elbow. I am **hooked on chocolate**. I crave it, and nothing else will do."

  –Ann Landers

- **"Hucklebears,"** milk chocolate bears filled with huckleberry cordial and whole huckleberries, won the Domestic Candy Award in the 13th Annual Product Awards Competition, sponsored by the National Association for the Specialty Food Trade. Said creator Louise "Cookie" Sevier, "I'm a chocoholic. Chocolate is so popular right now. And the combination of chocolate and huckleberries is superb."

- "We're a lot more **in touch with chocolate now**," says Alice Medrich of Coclat in Berkeley, California (*Chocolatier*, 1984). "It's an affordable luxury and somewhat of a sinful pleasure. I adore it any time of day, as long as it's not early in the morning. But once I get home in the evening, and I'm not wearing any clothes with chocolate ON them or IN them, I'm really ready to indulge."

- Chocolate artist Elaine Gonzalez asks, "Breathes there a man, woman, or child who has not lusted after it, devoured it, and moments later dreamed of it still? Chocolate is, quite frankly, **it**."

- Gertrude Parke, author of *The Big CHOCOLATE Cookbook* (A & W Visual Library, 1968), shares her nightmare: "Picture, if you can bear it, **life without chocolate**. Imagine existence without those beguiling chocolate desserts, those luscious candies, sauces, and syrups, all of which add charm and flavor to our daily fare, and the lack of which would form an intolerable privation."

- **Madame Chocolate** has observed that, "Chocolate makes us wicked, guilty, sinful, healthy, chic, happy."

- "After a nice meal, if I don't have a little chocolate sweet, the **meal isn't complete**."

  –Brad George, self-admitted chocoholic, quoted
  in the *Boston Globe* (February 10, 1985)

- **Montezuma,** Mexican Emperor of the Aztec Indians, is the first recorded chocoholic. He is said to have had 50 cups of "chocolatl" each day, serving another 2,000 to his royal household. He always had chocolate before going into his extensive harem–giving fuel to the aphrodisiac theory of chocolate.

- Fashion model **Margo Moore,** who calls herself a chocoholic since childhood, reminisces (in "Choc Talk"): "Of course, I was never allowed to have chocolate. High-fashion models, when I started modeling, were all skin and bones, but I sneaked it. I switched it around; I ate my dessert in the morning for breakfast. But I only ate only dark chocolate. That's the closest to base chocolate. Real chocolate, you know, is dark and bitter. As it gets sweeter and lighter, it's more caloric."

- ### "Ode to Chocolate"

Out of the lava darkness
Little bean of melting gladness
Once filled golden Aztec cups
Now blossoms in my mouth:
CHOCOLATE!

Elixir of the gods
Sweet, fragrant, silky
Tongue-touching:
CHOCOLATE!

Brown dark glorious soil-color
Inkling of sweet kisses
and fat bronze hugs
from a smiling black earthmother:
CHOCOLATE!

Lips lick up syrupy warmth
Liquid slips into cool milk.
Icing slaps on a cake
Candy bar rests in a foil wrapper
Nuggets wiggle in a bag
Blocks stack in a barrel
Truffles sit in a shiny box

Shells show in a glass case
Summer chocolate whitely bleaches
And bark sparkles with almonds:
CHOCOLATE!

At last I am lost in chocolate
Bathed in its delectable caress
Melting in a mocha madness
A cocoa climax
CHOCOLATE!

–Arlene G. Cohen, East Islip, New York (*Chocolate News,* Sept./Oct. 1981)

- Adrianne Marcus, author of *The Chocolate Bible* (G.P. Putnam, 1979), explains her **obsession** with chocolate in terms of "the remembrance of chocolates past. Each of us has known such moments of orgiastic anticipation, our senses focused at their finest, when control is irrevocably abandoned. Then the tongue possesses, is possessed by, what it most desires: the warmth, liquid melting of thick, dark chocolate." When she dies, Marcus declares, she's not going to be embalmed–"I'm going to be dipped."

- "I love good chocolate. I'm most tempted around 2 p.m. I'll be walking back and forth in the plant (Aphrodite: Confections of Love, in Huntington Beach, California) eyeing the candy-making . . . particularly the caramel-filled types . . . and I just go crazy. I'll grab a turtle or a Grand Marnier truffle. Now, that's the **pause that truly refreshes**."

    –Gloria Levine in *Chocolatier*'s Premier Issue

- At the age of 69 Paul Lawrence, a healthy lifelong chocoholic, wrote a health book titled *In Praise of Chocolate* (San Anselmo, California: Pal Press).

- **Chocolate quiz:**

    1. Do you get withdrawal symptoms if you don't fulfill your daily chocolate quota?
    2. Do you take two chocolates and go to bed when you feel a cold coming on?

3. Do you put chocolate in the freezer so you won't eat it, and then discover that it can taste even better frozen?
4. Do you drool thinking of (choco-)holidays?
5. Do you bypass meals, then "snack" on chocolate?
6. Do you have a morbid fear of an allergy to chocolate that preoccupies your mind?
7. Do you have dreams about drowning in a sea of chocolate?
8. Do you fantasize about being sculpted in chocolate?
9. Do you like to participate in Chocolate Quizzes?
10. Do you realize you have lots of company . . . if you answered "yes" to any (all?) of these questions?!

- Professor Susan Schiffman of Duke University Medical Center has been working on the notion of a **spray** that would fill cravings for flavors and aromas. She states, "It's the same process that (artificial-flavor makers) use. I found that overweight people want more taste and smell than thinner people, so I set out to give them that without the calories. If they can't live without the taste of chocolate or potato chips, they can spray this to their hearts' content."

- Dallas Alice of Rockville, Maryland, has a **T-shirt** proclaiming: "I think, talk, breathe, taste, eat, bite, devour, consume, swallow, touch, lick, suck, chew, feel, nibble, use, abuse, crave, prefer, require, request, handle, grab, snatch, steal, seek, hunt, find, hog, test, pick, choose, worship, idolize, adore, honor, enjoy, know, buy, collect, gather, accept, digest, understand, cook, bake, make, desire, produce, sneak, fancy, mooch, procure, ravish, glorify, serve, recommend, salute, respect, protect, support, welcome, suggest, order, demand, select, locate, demolish, gobble, want, need, and love anything and everything CHOCOLATE."

- Consumer Guide's *The Perfect Chocolate Dessert* (Publications International, 1981) discusses **taste associations** with chocolate: "Is there a more heavenly dessert on earth than exquisitely rich, satiny chocolate mousse? What sensual pleasure can compare with a brandy-kissed chocolate truffle melting on the tongue?"

- Consider: Healthy human beings have a "normal" temperature of 98.6° Fahrenheit–which is the same **temperature** as that of the melting point of cocoa butter.

- "Oh, it's a **terrible thing,** loving chocolate. I used to hide it from my kids. Honey, I think my mother's milk was chocolate. And I never wanted to be weaned!"

  > –A 67-year-old Sherman Oaks, California, woman at Chocolate Expo, quoted in the *Los Angeles Times*, May 15, 1983

- "I achieve (the) **zenith of ecstasy** when a perfect eclair, ridged with rich chocolate fudge, is presented to me, and as I allow the fork to pierce the delicate golden shell, a rewarding river of silken custard is revealed. The Ultimate Brownie is my goal: fudgy in the middle, cake-like on top. A bittersweet chocolate cake is not to be denied, of course–the fondant on the outside giving way to layer after layer of moist, dense chocolate cake inside–beauty in its purest form."

  > –Judith Lewis, "A Dieter's Dilemma," in *Chocolatier*'s Premier Issue

- Honey and Larry **Zisman** chronicle these *Chocolate Fantasies*: chocolate bedtime pillows, chocolate fingernails, an all-chocolate home shopping TV network, chocolate leaves, chocolate necktie, an edible chocolate book, chocolate straws, a Chocolate Emergency Service with 24-hour service, the banning of Chocoholics Anonymous, chocolate shaving cream, a discovery that "copious consumption of chocolate leads to permanent weight loss," an addition to the Declaration of Independence about our unalienable rights to "Life, Liberty, and the Pursuit of Chocolate," changing the United Nations symbol to a chocolate chip, chocolate spigots, chocolate hot tubs, a vacation at Club Choc, a process to transform spinach into chocolate having the "Hershey Touch" (the ability to turn anything you touch into chocolate), chocolate toothpaste, going to a chocotorium, chocolate-based paint, chocolate telephones, a transcontinental chocolate pipeline, chocolate sleep inducers, portable intravenous chocolate, and chocolate that glows in the dark.

CHOCOLATE FEASTS

- "**All I eat is chocolate** now. I start out the day with a handful of chocolate-covered macadamia nuts and tea. At 10 a.m. it's a Grand Marnier truffle, 11:30 amaretto cappuccino truffle, and a salad and chocolate for dinner. I went through the health food thing. It was sheer trauma. Now I eat whatever I want, and I'm happy."

  –Sara Bancroft, quoted in the *Los Angeles Times*, May 15, 1983

- The famous London coffee house where people used to gather for chocolate "in the Spanish style" in 1674 was named **"At the Coffee Mill and Tobacco Roll."**

- **Better Homes and Gardens'** *Chocolate* (Meredith Corporation, 1984) encourages feasting on the following: chocolate strawberry shortcake, feathery fudge cake, banana-split cake, chocolate cake roll a la mode, chocolate fruitcake, two-tone clover cookies, tri-level brownies, chocolate-dipped fondant, marble-top chocolate-rum pie, chocolate marble pumpkin pie, chocolate puff pastry, chocolate-cinnamon meringue torte, chocolate chip-coffee cheesecake, creme de menthe cheesecake, chocolate souffle, chocolate Irish coffee ice cream, ice cream snowball pie, raspberry-brownie baked Alaska, mocha mousse, chocolate-nutmeg bavarian, chocolate-caramel popcorn, chocolate bismarcks, chocolate grasshoppers, and chocolate creme liqueur.

- Instead of a traditional chocolate cake for a crowd, try a huge **brownie sheet cake**. Marriott Food Services suggests making two, putting frosting between them, and a message on top. Of course you can add ice cream, sauce, and chocolate sprinkles, too!

- "**Businessmen** keep candy bars at hand to fight fatigue at the end of a long grueling day; their office and factory workers follow suit, finding that chocolate raises their blood-sugar level, and so helps them to stay alert during that afternoon slump," says chocolate cookbook author Gertrude Parke.

- If you crave chocolate for breakfast, try the **"Chocolate Banana Nut Loaf"** that Chef Martin Johner of the Culinary Institute of New York has devised in his book *Mountains of Chocolate* (Irena Chalmers, 1981).

- Harry Levene of London has a **chocolate bar wrapper** collection of nearly 50,000 kinds from 93 countries. Germany leads, with 7,778 wrappers from 347 brands, followed by Spain with 145 brands. His vote for the best chocolate is Switzerland; for the worst–Rumania, closely followed by Bulgaria, Yugoslavia, and Costa Rica. Imagine what fun he had testing all those candy bars!

- The 27-foot-long table featured at Mohonk Mountain's **"Chocolate Binge"** included the following: chocolate soufflés, Black Forest Cake, eclairs, cream puffs and tarts, chocolate cream cakes, chocolate cheesecake, chocolate chiffon pies, chocolate croquembouche, Dobosh tortes, German chocolate cakes, Boston Cream Pie, chocolate chip cookies, and chocolate fudge brownies. A ton of chocolate was reportedly consumed by 360 guests in three days–the equivalent of an annual per capita rate of about 700 pounds!

- You can get a 15-lb, 2-1/2-foot-in-diameter **chocolate chip cookie** delivered to you in the New York City area by Captain Cookie, on request–it will only cost you $150!

- When 700 chocoholics participated in the one-week **chocolate cruise** to Alaska in August of 1984, "A Chocolate Celebration on the Sun Princess," they consumed nearly a ton of chocolate. Needless to say, they had a "Bon Bon Voyage."

- The sixteenth century chocolate craze inspired silversmiths and porcelain manufacturers to produce chocolate pots and chocolate

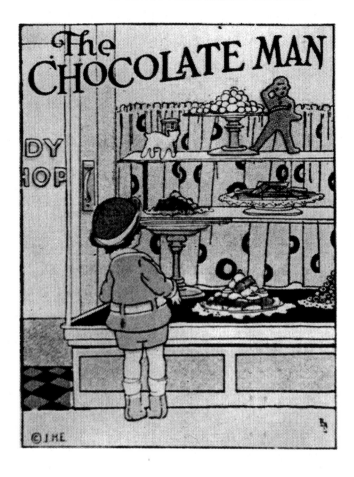

cups. Many of those exquisite **chocolate serving pieces** are exhibited in museums throughout Europe. Austria had the most elaborate designs, fashioned in Baroque style, while Madame de Pompadour (1721-1764), mistress to Louis XV of France, is reputed to have owned the most expensive porcelain set ever made.

- Barbara Myers' *Chocolate, Chocolate, Chocolate* (Penguin, 1983) gives directions for making **chocolate scrolls, shavings, lace, and sprinkles**, as well as garnishes.

- "There's definitely a new **chocolate snob** emerging. Last year people would ask me, 'What's a truffle?' Now they ask, 'Who makes your truffles?' "

  –Meagan O'Meara of San Francisco's Chocolate Heaven (quoted in *Newsweek,* April 4, 1983)

- Karl Bissinger of St. Louis operates a popular one-pound **"Confection of the Month"** program for $250 per year. October, for example, features the Bissinger Bear Claws, a secret cluster of caramel, pecans, and chocolate.

- "The entire over-the-counter candy bar industry is 95 percent milk chocolate. People are weaned on it. Dark chocolate is a **connoisseur's chocolate**–more tasty, richer. As a result, a person who wants that will never buy milk."

  –Joe Foscaldo, Marketing Manager for Phillips Candy House (quoted in *Boston Globe*)

- *The Chocolate Cookbook* (Bobbs-Merrill, 1973) by **Juliette Elkon** offers feasting on apricot or tangerine upside-down chocolate cake, chocolate applesauce cake, bran brownies, chocolate pancakes and doughnuts, chocolate popovers, glazed chocolate chip bread, steamed chocolate date pudding, chocolate caramel flan, cherry chocolate fool, raspberry chocolate charlotte, almond chocolate soufflé, minted chocolate fudge, chocolate peanut brittle, plus many suggestions for chocolate decorations.

- **Chocolate Emotions, Ltd.** of New York City is available to fulfill your chocolate emotional needs on 48 hours' notice. Their message: "Give us a call and we'll provide love, lust, desire, passion, or ecstasy."

- When Michel Richard of Los Angeles gave **"An Evening of Chocolate,"** he made lots of chocolate desserts, including: almond chocolate mousse cake layered with almond meringue and wrapped in a thin layer of chocolate, chocolate cake with praline

cream, chocolate brownies laced with Grand Marnier, and hazelnut chocolate sponge cake soaked in rum.

–cited in *Chocolatier*'s Premier Issue

- It's been figured out that if you are a 35-year-old lifetime member of **Fanny Farmer**'s Chocolate-of-the-Month Club, you'll be
getting nearly 450 pounds of chocolate! To burn up the 1.1 million calories, some options include jogging from New York to
Chicago 11 times, walking nonstop for 15 months, or bike riding
roundtrip from New York to Melbourne, Australia.

- On the subject of **"Fasting from Chocolate in Lent,"** Daniel
Concuna published the following statement in Venice in 1748:
"Consumers are, without the help of casuists, troubled themselves and afflicted, when in Lent they empty chocolate cups . . .
Excited on the one hand by the pungent cravings of the throat to
moisten it, reproved on the other by breaking their fast, they
experience grave remourses of conscience, and, with consciences
agitated and torn with drinking the sweet beverage, they sin . . .
Under the guidance of these skillful theologians, the remorse
aroused by natural and Divine light being blunted, Christians
drink joyfully."

- For millions of Americans, according to *Time* magazine (July 12,
1982), "The product of the cocoa bean is not so much a feast as a
fix."

- "Well-made chocolate is such a noble invention that it, rather
than nectar and ambrosia, should be known as the **food of the
gods.**"

–Dr. Bachot (1685), physician of Queen
Maria-Therese of Austria

- Dutch children are brought up with **"bagelslag,"** chocolate shot
(jimmies or sprinkles) sprinkled on slices of bread or Holland
rusks; it's a standard daily breakfast, lunch, and snack specialty.

- In a custom dating back to the seventeenth century, Chocolateria
San Gines in Madrid is open for **hot chocolate** only from 5-10

a.m., then again from 5-10 p.m., to accommodate workers' and families' schedules. For 100 years the shop has been a gathering place for laborers, shoppers, school children, and friends. Only hot chocolate and churros (a form of fried dough) are served.

▪ Some **international classics** featuring chocolate include these:

Austria–Sachertorte
Bavaria–Chocolate crepes
Brazil–Hot chocolate
England–English toffee
France–Chocolate Mousse
Germany–German chocolate cake
Greece–Chocolate-nut candy
Hungary–Black Forest Cake
Israel–Cocoa Cheesecake
Italy–Chocolate Toronne
Mexico–Mole
Netherlands–Cocoa brittle
Switzerland–Chocolate fondue
United States–Chocolate chip cookies, brownies, fudge

▪ David Hoffman, author of *The Joy of Pigging Out*, conducts seminars on where to go, how to dress, what to eat, and other secrets of his "pig out" diet.

▪ "Chocolate isn't just candy anymore. It's **life style**."

–*Advertising Age* (September 9, 1984)

▪ Mexicans use a special wooden beater, called a **"molinillo,"** to froth up hot chocolate. Place the beater in the chocolate, rub it between both hands until the proper consistency is reached, then guzzle.

▪ *A Tale of Two Cities*, by Charles Dickens (1859) describes this feast:

Monseigneur, one of the great lords in power at the Court, held his fortnightly reception in his grand hotel in Paris. Monseigneur was in his inner room, his sanctuary of sanctuaries, the Holiest of Holiests to the crowd of worshippers in the suite of rooms without. Monseigneur was about to take his chocolate. Monseigneur could swallow a great many things with ease, and was by some few sullen minds supposed to be rather rapidly swallowing France; but, his morning's chocolate could not so much as get into the throat of Monseigneur without the aid of four strong men besides the cook.

Yes. It took four men, all four a-blaze with gorgeous decoration, and the chief of them was unable to exist with fewer than two gold watches in his pocket, emulative of the noble and chaste fashion set by Monseigneur, to conduct the happy chocolate to Monseigneur's lips. Once lacquey carried the chocolate-pot into the sacred presence; a second milled and frothed the chocolate with the little instrument he bore for that function; a third presented the favoured napkin; a fourth (he of the two gold watches) poured the chocolate out. It was impossible for Monseigneur to dispense with one of these attendants on the chocolate and hold his high place under the admiring Heavens. Deep would have been the blot upon his escutcheon if his chocolate had been ignobly waited on by only three men; he must have died of two.

- Bernal Diaz de Castillo, who was present at one of **Montezuma's feasts**, reported that 50 golden goblets of chocolate were served to guests of the banquet, while another 2,000 were served to the guards and attendants.

- Some of the most festive dinners use chocolate as a **mystery ingredient** in savory sauces that blend well with meats and poultry-like mole sauce.

- "Chocolate, thy mystique is everywhere. The eating of chocolate, once a very quiet, private matter, now has gone **public** in a big way."

  –Mary Alice Kellogg, *Signature* (February 1983)

- One of the highlights of Uncommon Boston's chocolate tour of the city is at **Rebecca's Restaurant** on Charles Street: silver platters brimming with truffles, chocolate-covered strawberries, chocolate mousse cups, a torte, and three cakes: concord, mousse, and devil's food.

- There are **regional differences** in the United States in chocolate preferences. Southwesterners like "mole" (spicy chocolate dressing for poultry); Appalachians put it on biscuits for breakfast; Southerners like Mississippi Mud; while East and West coasters are most prone to purchasing "designer chocolates."

- **"The Spanish ladies of the New World,** it is said, carried their love for chocolate to such a degree that, not content with partaking of it several times a day, they had it sometimes carried after them to church."

  –Brillat-Savarin, "Physiologie du Gout"

- The week between Christmas and New Year's is known in France as **"la treve des confiseurs"** (the confectioners' truce), when affairs of state are suspended so citizens can indulge themselves in serious chocolate-feasting.

- According to the 1880 publication "The Manufacture of Chocolate and Cocoa" by J. S. Fry and Sons, "The **virulently narcotic cocoa leaf of Peru** is chewed by natives of the west coast of South America."

- **World-wide chocolate consumption** per capita:

Austria	11.6 lbs/person/year
Belgium	13.6
England	15.4
Sweden	11.6
Switzerland	22
United States	10
West Germany	13.8

- "As a newly christened **Yuppie,**" Hilary DeVries (*Christian Science Monitor,* November 11, 1984) recognizes she's expected to be "busy patronizing those restaurants displaying a requisite amount of ferns, brass, and marble, where I never eat macaroni and cheese or tuna on white. I am too busy stoking up on sushi, gravlax, and gourmet chocolates."

CHOCOLATE LOVE

- The Jesuit priest **Acosta** claimed that if the monks of his acquaintance had been prohibited from drinking chocolate, "the scandal with which the holy order has been branded might have proved groundless."

- The legend about chocolate being an **aphrodisiac** dates from Emperor Montezuma of Mexico's habit in the 1500s of drinking several full goblets of "chocolatl" before entering his harem.

- **Aphrodite Confections of Love**, located in Huntington Beach, California, specializes in the "3 Ts" of chocolate: turtles, truffles, and toffee.

- Perugina's **"Baci,"** the Italian word for "kisses," were named in honor of a love affair in the 1930s between Giovani Buitoni and an older, married woman. Their only means of communication was love messages via hand-wrapped chocolates, which Buitoni commemorated after his love's death.

- **Erma Bombeck** reports in her syndicated newspaper column ("At Wit's End," February 14, 1985) that after telling her husband about chocolate being an aphrodisiac, she hated to consider "what would happen if someone gave me a three-pound box of chocolate creams."

- Maida Heatter, who has been referred to as "The First Lady of American Desserts," keeps returning to **brownies** as a favorite. She explains that brownies were a Cupid's Arrow to her marriage; the recipe in her first book was the key to her husband

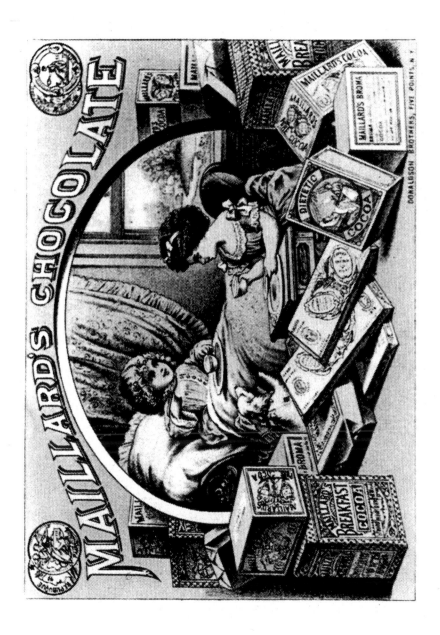

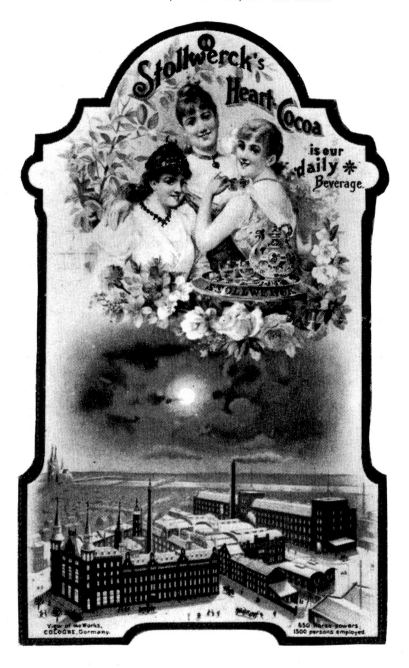

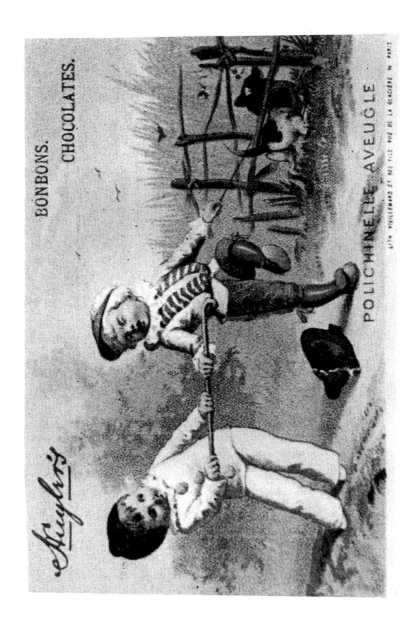

BONBONS.

CHOCOLATES.

POLICHINELLE AVEUGLE

183

Ralph's heart. He tells the story: "I was at a party in Miami and Maida came around serving these brownies. I took one bite and thought, 'This is wonderful. I wonder what else she can do.' "

–quoted in *Christian Science Monitor* (November 6, 1985)

- **Richard Cadbury**, son of the founder of Cadbury, Ltd., invented the heart-shaped Valentine's Day candy box in 1861.

- **Casanova**, the legendary Italian adventurer and lover, reportedly claimed to use chocolate as often as champagne as a tool for seduction. (This apparently also was true of the Marquis de Sade!)

- It has been said that the best way to test a relationship is to have a **"courtchip."**

- Aloysius **Ferronius**, a Jesuit priest, wrote this ode to the chocolate tree, dedicated to Cardinal Francis Maria Brancaccio of the Vatican, in 1664:

  O tree, born in far off lands,
  Price of Mexico's shores,
  Rich with a heavenly nectar
  That will conquer all who taste it.

  To thee let every tree pay homage,
  And every flower bow its head in praise
  The wreath of the laurel crowns you; the oak, the alder,
  And the precious cedar proclaim your triumph.

  Some say you lived in Eden with Adam
  And that he carried you with him when he fled.
  And from thence you journeyed to the Indes
  Where you prospered in the hospitable soil,
  And your trunk burgeoned with
  The bounty of your noble seeds.

  And you another gift of Bacchus,
  Famed for his free-flowing wines?
  No–the fruits of Crete and Massica
  Bring not the glory you do to your native land.

For you are a fresh shower that bedews the heart,
The fountain of the poet's gentle spirit.
O sweet liquor sent from the stars.
Surely you must be the drink of the gods!

- "Today, the **gift** of chocolate is associated with affection, love and tender feelings toward a special person. Chocolate molds of every description result in imaginative candies, bonbons and similar treats."

    –Bo Niles, *Country Living* (February 1983)

- According to Nestle's Study of "The Boxed Chocolate Market," nearly 50% of **chocolates purchased as gifts** are reported to be bought at specialty candy shops.

- Question: Do you think that since chocolate has been a traditional Valentine's Day gift for years that there is a historical or genuine link between love and chocolate–that chocolate is the **gift of love?** Answer (Maxwell Glen and Cody Shearer, journalists): "Anthropologists have been asking the same question for years. Nonetheless, their research isn't conclusive. So far, however, they've proved links between love and, among other things, adultery, attempted assassination and the arms race. Chocolate would be a positive addition to the list–at least it's only fattening."

- This Swiss poem dates to the nineteenth century:

    Young Jacob holds a pistol in his hand,
    And says, "I'll kill myself my dear Susanne,
    Unless you say you'll marry me as planned."
    She stares, aghast, as the cool tempered man
    Serenely holds the pistol to his head.
    The girl cries, "Stop!" But Jacob seems upset:
    The trigger's pulled . . .
       Instead of dropping dead,
    He eats the **gun**: it's only chocolate!
    He chuckles as he chews it like a gangster.
    No wonder she won't wed this foolish prankster.

- Hershey Food Corporation produces 20-25 million **Hershey Kisses** each day; don't you wonder how that stacks up against the daily average for "real" kisses?

- The giving of chocolates carries with it an assumption of expectation of **intimacy**. It is to melt in the mouth of the recipient, and intoxicate the senses. Chocolate, in both essence and mythology, is an aphrodisiac. It is a fond declaration of love, and a plea for its reciprocation."

–Chris Savage King

- In **Japan**, girls give chocolates to boys on Valentine's Day, not the other way around. A chocolate manufacturer's survey of 15,000 females in Tokyo, ranging in age from 10 to 40, found 80% of them planning to give presents to men. Of $1.67 billion worth of Japanese chocolate sales in 1984, 10% took place during the first two weeks in February. There are three types of chocolate-giving:
  1. "Raby," the Japanese equivalent of "love," is the most common–chocolates given to boyfriends and crushes.
  2. Girls with no boyfriends get "dojo-choco," sympathy chocolate, from parents and girlfriends, as do boys who wouldn't otherwise get anything.
  3. Obligation chocolate, "giri-choco," is given to male teachers and bosses to show loyalty.

–*Christian Science Monitor* (February 11, 1985)

- Saying it is in the **"Large Kiss Business,"** Harry London's of North Canton, Ohio, features a 4-lb Super Kiss, "Hot Lips," L-O-V-E letters in chocolate, the "Ultimate Kiss," and of course chocolate hearts.

- **Lindt** spent $2 million in 1984 to capture the "romance" of its products; it expects $15 million in sales this year.

- "**Lovers** always want the biggest and the best. The biggest velour heart filled with all Perugina. The box itself is all wrapped in hearts and red and gold paper. The $22 one-pounders are for girlfriends and mothers. Wives is another story . . . "

–Joe Matana, Manager of Dairy Fresh Candies
in Boston (quoted in the *Boston Globe*)

- According to Joan Steuer, editor of *Chocolatier*, "**Ninety-eight percent** of the country loves chocolate, and the other 2% are either allergic or won't admit it because they're closet chocophiles."

- "If there is a single food in this country that arouses **passionate devotion** to the Nth degree, chocolate has to be well up there in the running for first-place honors."

–Betsy Balsley of the *Los Angeles Times*

- **Phenylethylamine**, a mood-altering chemical present in chocolate, has been documented as helping to cure a broken heart.

- Alan Winecour, a tour guide for Uncommon Boston, posits (in the *Boston Globe*, February 10, 1985) that "chocolate certainly is a **reflection** of affection and love."

- In 1662, royal physician **Henry Stubbe** dubbed chocolate, "The Indian Nectar," and expounded on its powers to incite Venus: "As chocolate provokes other Evacuations through the several Emunctories of the body, so it doth that of seed, and becomes provocative to lust upon no other account than that it begets good blood."

- Chocolate is the #1 best-selling candy for **Valentine's Day**. Ask any sweets emporium vendor! Phyllis Hanes, staff writer of the *Christian Science Monitor* (2/4/87) reminds us that, "To our ancestors, chocolate was an exotic luxury, like caviar and truffles are today. At times it was reported to cost as much as $300 an ounce. . . . Chocolate is an emotional food associated with warmth, sweetness, and contentment–as symbolized by the heart-shaped Valentine's Day box.

CHOCOLATE PARTIES

- For a safari party, dip **animal crackers** in chocolate, then use to decorate cakes and party favors.

- For your next **beach** outing, be sure to bring along cocoa butter to lather on everyone; not only does it melt on contact with your skin, but the whole crowd will smell deliciously of chocolate!

- "Venus. Thoughts thought After a **Bridge Party**"

> Women are ethereal beings,
>   subsisting entirely on
>   chocolate marshmallow nut
>   sundaes and cantaloupe,
> But they open up a package
>   of cigarettes like a lioness
>   opening up an antelope.

–Ogden Nash

- Hyatt Regency Hotels squeeze in games of **"CACAO"** between chocolate meals at their chocolate "getaway" packages–it's BINGO, played with cocoa beans.

- For a teacher friend's 40th birthday, we gave him the following **candy bar** collection and comments: "Skip, now that you're at the SUMMIT of life, we want to have a few CHUCKLES to BOLSTER your ego. As you now GO AHEAD with (the school superintendent and his assistant) as the 3 MUSKETEERS of education along the MILKY WAY of learning, we wish you a BIT-O-HONEY. There will be MOUNDS of decisions: whether to earn $100,000 (BAR) and strut along 5th AVENUE, or ZERO and stay with your SUGAR BABIES. If you left, your students couldn't get their SNICKERS watching MR. GOODBAR pick and eat his own GOOBERS. Both NOW OR LATER it's time you learn to control your BUTTERFINGER over Carol's POM POMS. But, when you put your SMOOOOTH N' JUICY WHATCHAMACALLIT TWIX her legs, it always makes her STARBURST. The combination of your CHUNKY TOOTSIE

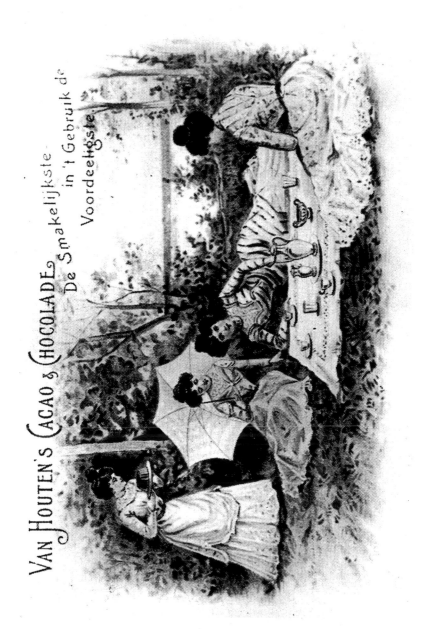

VAN HOUTEN'S CACAO & CHOCOLADE
De Smakelijkste -
in 't Gebruik de
Voordeeligste

ROLL and her WHOPPERS make for GOOD AND PLENTY fun times! So, stick with the MARATHON–we all think you're fun, and pretty SPECIAL.

- **Chocolate Bake-Offs** are great fun: send invitations to your guests (on chocolate-decorated stationery) to bring their best/favorite chocolate creations. Here are some rules for running the contest:
    1. Determine a numerical scale, such as 1 to 10 or 1 to 100
    2. You'll want to taste the outside, the inside, and any fillings and/or garnishes
    3. Evaluate overall appearance
    4. Consider flavor, texture, and moisture
    Winners get all the leftovers–if there are any!

- Consider having your next party **chocolate-catered**: specialists can set you up with chocolate placecards, chocolate centerpieces, chocolate plates and utensils, chocolate decorations–all, of course, to be eaten by you and your guests.

- Lee Gelfond, a Beverly Hills caterer, made 125 **chocolate chickens** for one of Henry ("The Fonz") Winkler's parties.

- Your **Chocolate Dessert Party** is guaranteed to be an orgy of delights. Set up, in different rooms, any of the following combinations: chocolate soufflé, chocolate cheesecake, chocolate cupcakes, chocolate fudge, chocolate mousse, chocolate liqueurs, chocolate ice cream with fudge sauce, chocolate cookies, etc.

- The **Chocolate Experience** of Hillsdale, New Jersey, plans and performs your birthday, annual meeting, and/or whatever chocolate extravagant excuse you'd like for celebration.

- As the frequenting of coffee houses was passing from the fashionable to the populace in the mid-seventeenth century, **chocolate houses** for the "elite" opened in major cities like London and Amsterdam. As a new, costly, and delicious item, chocolate became an ideal favorite of the elegant and refined.

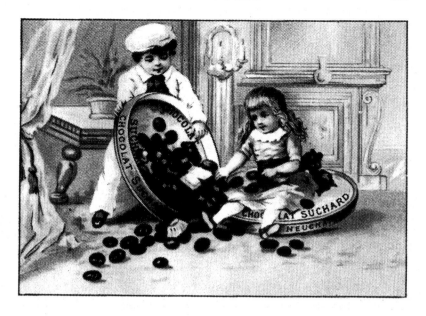

- **Chocolate liqueurs** provide a pleasant ending to a dinner, or can be a whole reason for a get-together in themselves. While creme de cacao is the most popular, you might also try chocolate cordial combinations with fruit, nuts, coconut, coffee, spices, and cream. They can all be served plain, in coffee, or as ice cream topping.

- Audrey Ellis has put together "a glorious selection of chocolate recipes for candy, cakes, cookies, puddings, and pies" in her *Chocolate Lovers Cookbook* (Exeter, 1984). Whip some up for your next chocolate excuse, and leave the book out so guests can see the marvelous mouthwatering color photos.

- **Chocolate mousse,** originally called "chocolate mayonnaise," was invented by the French painter Henri de Toulouse-Lautrec who, in the mid-1880s, celebrated the bohemian life of fellow Montmartre entertainers and artists.

- You should see the **chocolate orgy**/media blitz party we're planning with the publication of this book!

- **Chocolate services** have long been indications of status produced by silversmiths and porcelain manufacturers like Limoges. The most expensive chocolate service created is said to have belonged to Madame de Pompadour.

- British youngsters often serve **chocolate soup** on special occasions: combine 1/4 cup milk, 3 Tablespoons sugar, 1 teaspoon vanilla, and 2 Tablespoons cocoa to a paste; slowly add 2 cups of milk and 1 cup of heavy cream and 2 egg yolks; heat until blended and thick. Serve with scones or graham crackers.

- How about organizing a **Chocolate Tasting?** It's best to test together chocolates with similar traits, such as fillings, country of origin, chocolate color and/or texture, truffles, etc. Proceed as you would for a wine tasting, slowly and discriminatingly, clearing the palate between tastings with some wine, cognac, or plain water.

- In the German tradition of celebrating the tenth month of the year, try a variation and hold a **"Choctoberfest"**!

- A traditional European tradition at **Christmas** is wrapping chocolate ornaments, then hanging them on the Christmas tree.

- **Christmastime in Germany** often features events where chocolate cookies are served: Schokoladen Kringel (chocolate rings, often covered with sugar pearls), Lebkuchen (spicy pastry dough coated with chocolate), Spitzkuchen (jam-filled chocolate-coated pyramids), and Elisen (hazelnut pastry covered with a chocolate-sugar icing).

- Charbonnel et Walker tell the story of the New York hostess who found her **dinner chocolate-mint supply** getting low, so she flew her chauffeur to London to replenish it.

- Spread a **"Viennese Table"**: combinations of fruits, cheeses, pastries, chocolates, and liqueurs in chocolate cups.

- Judith Elkon (*The Chocolate Cookbook*, Bobbs-Merrill, 1973) suggests a **do-it-yourself dessert** of chocolate fondue with any combinations of these dippers: seedless green grapes, apple slices or wedges, banana chunks or slices, pear wedges, stemmed cherries, tangerine sections, dried apricots, prunes, marshmallows, dates, candied orange rind, butter cookies, toasted pound cake strips, pretzels, rolled cookies, ladyfingers, flat mints, and anything else you'd like to dip in chocolate.

▪ **Dreams Come True** out of Pittsburgh gained fame in chocolate circles for a chocolate nose it created a few years ago as a party request. Aly Adams, President, plans surprises, events, retirements, and unusual gifts for individuals and people in business.

▪ To celebrate the **engagement announcement** of their colleague Mark Simmons to Sissy Doty, William Hamilton and Associates of Nashville honored them with a chocolate and champagne party.

▪ Many chocolate companies allow **factory tours**. If you've wondered about the manufacturing process, here is a description of one: Van Leer Chocolate Corporation of Jersey City, New Jersey.

"After delivery at the plant, cocoa beans are checked for quality, flavor, color, and cleanliness by the company's trained laboratory staff. When approved, the beans are pneumatically conveyed to the roaster, where, with the proper temperature and timing, they develop the rich brown chocolate color and flavor. Next step is the cracker-fanner, where the shells are removed from the nibs (the meat of the cocoa bean.) The nibs are crushed and ground, and the result is the unsweetened chocolate known in the trade as liquor chocolate.

Liquor chocolate goes into the paste mixers, where liquid and dry ingredients are blended into a paste. A specially designed steel conveying system moves the paste to heavy five-roll refiners to be ground to a fine velvety-smooth consistency. After refining, the chocolate is mixed–or conched–until the flavor and viscosity are approved by the lab. It is then pumped into storage tanks, and from there into drums, pails, or tank trucks, holding up to 40,000 pounds of liquid chocolate, for delivery to our bulk customers.

In another part of the plant, chocolate is molded into bars for use by confectioners and ice cream makers. This chocolate is piped overhead through the plant to the tempering machine; then it is automatically weighed into trays to move slowly through the cooling tunnel. One hour later, the solidly formed bars are encased in plastic bags, packed in cartons, and taken by forklift truck to the temperature-controlled warehouse.

From the time the raw materials are received at the plant until the finished products are ready for delivery, constant testing is the rule.

Regularly throughout manufacture, batches are checked for flavor, color, fineness, viscosity. In addition, every batch is tested in our own microbiology lab and sent out for inspection to independent bacteriology labs.''

- When *Chocolatier* magazine ran tests to discover what **flavors** go best with chocolate (Vol 1, #6, 1985), raspberry and orange came out on top, with apricot and mocha also emerging as popular choices. It also found these wines as good chocolate accompaniments: Essensia (orange muscat), Elysium (black muscat), Schramsberg (a sparkling wine), Cabernet Sauvignon (full-bodied red), Zinfandel (heavy, rich wine with ripe fruit overtones), and Prager (ruby port).

- You could have your **invitations** to a chocolate event printed in the real thing: The Chocolate Letter in New York City does 30 words for $19.95, up to 90 words for $21.95.

- Did you hear the **joke** about Peppermint Patty having an affair with Mr. Goodbar? The result was Baby Ruth! See if you can make up any more at your next party . . .

- For friends' 25th wedding anniversary, we gave them, amongst other group gifts at the surprise party, **25 (Hershey) Kisses**. And a friend gave her chocoholic grandmother 100 of them recently for her centennial birthday.

- **Math problem** to try on your dinner guests: each cocoa tree has about 15-16 pods, with 25-50 cocoa beans in each pod. After the beans are dried, they weigh less than 2 oz each. If it takes about

400 dried cocoa beans to make a pound of chocolate liquor, and if we 236.6 million Americans (Statistical Abstracts, 1984) each consume about 10 pounds of chocolate per year, how many cocoa beans are needed to keep us stocked in chocolate each year?

- When Zubin **Mehta**, music director of the New York Philharmonic, gave his final performance on May 28, 1991, Great Performances caterers staged a post-concert champagne and dessert reception, with chocolate donated by Nestle.

- Chocolate Pix of Utica, New York, has just the party favor for you: individual **chocolate place cards** made into shapes of photos of the guest(s) of honor. Simply brush on a little confectioners' sugar and the image appears.

- Larry and Honey Zisman's *Chocolate Fantasies* includes some unusual **recipes** using chocolate, with ingredients like fruits (peaches, strawberries, nectarines, raspberries, oranges, pineapple, prunes, apricots, dates), cheese, applesauce, coconut, cola, mashed potato, zucchini, cognac, bourbon, cornflakes, tortillas, peanuts, and peanut butter.

- Apparently pianist **Rudolf Serkin** has admitted that he far more appreciates a box of fancy chocolates to a bottle of champagne after a performance.

- **Harriet Beecher Stowe** is said to have declared in 1869 that chocolate as considered a Spanish or French item, improper for American tables.

- In a tradition dating from the twelfth century, many Mexicans still **toast happiness** with hot, sweetened chocolate.

- **Top off** a French party with "Mousse au Chocolate"; a German one with a "Chocolate Kuchen"; Italian–"Chocolate Rum Cake"; Austrians like "Chocolate Sacher Torte"; "Chocolate Pudding" would be appropriate for a Dutch (treat) party; Swiss "Chocolate Fondue" is always fun; or try American "Chocolate Brownies" or "Chocolate Chip Cookies."

- Try a **"Truffle-Off"**: contestants assign a rate scale to at least a dozen samples each, and try to determine a winner. The best way to test truffles is to cut them in half so you can make distinctions about the centers and how they relate to the chocolate coating.

- In celebration of his book *O Dolce Mio* that he produced around photographs commissioned by Chiara Samugheo of Rome, Max Felchlin held a **"Vernissage"** on May 17, 1985, at his Vanini chocolate shop in Zurich. At 7 p.m. we 80 specially-invited guests were given an apertif and listened to a classical guitarist. Peter Ahrens, a well-known Swiss actor, read Goethe's "Prologue to Faust," and Max and his wife Suzanne Felchlin explained the background to the project and the pictures. Champagne, meat and fish pastries, pork pâté, and salad were but preludes to what became a standing ovation to the chocolate creations the chefs prepared for the celebration.

CHOCOLATE PROMOTIONS

- In celebration of its 150th anniversary in 1976, Suchard of Switzerland reproduced an **1898 advertisement** it had run of a youngster holding a box of its chocolates.

- A different kind of advertising gimmick was used in 1926 by a German chocolate manufacturer who decided to drop its candies from an **airplane** on a group of Berliners; the police, however, stopped the campaign when people complained about the chocolate barrage.

- The **art world** has been inspired by chocolate since its discovery in the New World. An early seventeenth century Latin frontispiece showed Neptune being handed a box of "Inda Chocolata" by an Indian maiden, and paintings of aristocracy often include a cup of chocolate. The eighteenth century brought the chocolate pot and chocolate service pieces. By the nineteenth century, Richard Cadbury had introduced the chocolate box, which has taken on forms ranging from the elaborate to the sentimental or romantic. And since the twentieth century, commercial art has

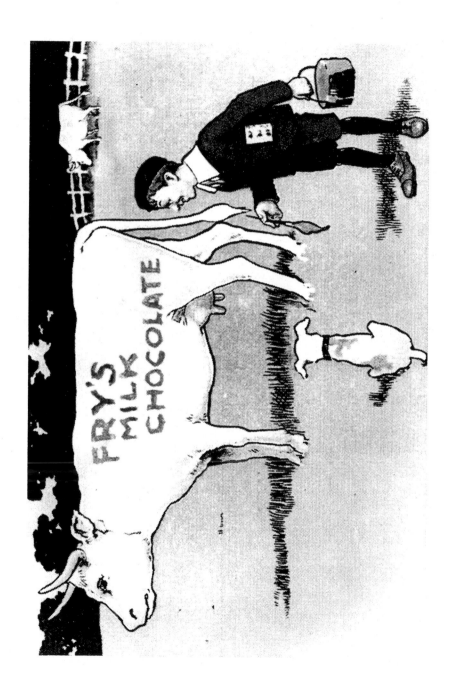

dominated, as many chocolate companies have produced their products in popular art forms.

- Book-of-the-Month Club commissioned Harbor Sweets to make exclusive **book-shaped** white and dark chocolates for their Holiday Gift Collection.

- Admission is free to the **Candy Americana Museum**–Wilbur Chocolate's Factory Candy Outlet in Lititz, Pennsylvania. Encouraging tourists to "relive the sweet past," the museum contains a large collection of antiques and old-time equipment used by our country's first candy makers, featuring all phases of the industry: manufacturing, processing, packaging, and advertising. A 1900 candy kitchen displays tools, molds, tins, chocolate porcelain pots, and wood and metal candy containers.

- Pulakos 926 Candies, in Erie, Pennsylvania, since 1904, runs a **candy school** for members of the chocolate industry.

- The United States Candy Industry recently launched a $500,000 Public Relations campaign under the motto that **"Candy is happiness."**

- The **Chocolate Bakery** in Northampton, Massachusetts, features chocolate truffles, cocoa bread, chocolate-covered nuts, brownies, and chocolate fortune cookies. Poetry readings and art and photographic exhibitions add further to attract customers.

- Jane Farmer, Director of the Chocolate Lovers Club, includes an updated **"Chocolate Calendar" listing** of chocolate events as a public service to *Chocolatier* magazine.

- With customers from Maine to Florida, Wisconsin to Texas, Van Leer Chocolate Corporation maintains a **"chocolate doctor"** who makes house calls or does telephone consultations from the company's Jersey City, New Jersey, office.

- William Frost Mobley, rare books and antiques collector/dealer, has a unique collection of more than 400 **chocolate ephemera** items in his Schoharie, New York, home. Collections can include chocolate cutouts, chocolate posters, chocolate containers, chocolate wrappers, etc.

- *Chocolate News*, "The World's Favorite Flavor Newsletter," encourages **"Choc Exchange,"** a classified ad forum for trades, offers, exchanges, and services.

- Stouffer Westchester (New York) Hotel and Nestle sponsored a **"Chocofrolic Weekend"** recently where participants learned how to make their own truffles, indulged in chocolate tastings, helped judge a chocolate scholarship competition, and danced to a Brown-and-White Sock Hop.

- Mohonk Mountain in New Paltz, New York, offered **"Chocolate Binge"** weekend packages from 1982-85. According to Carol Schimmer, Program Director, "We started in 1982 as the original Bingers, similar to freshmen in college. For four years we grew in knowledge and refined our tastes until we were able to graduate from Chocolate University in 1985. The program has now ended, and we're on to bigger and better things." The tradition at Mohonk continues to this day.

- Duncan Hines had a "Chocolate Lovers Sweepstakes" awarding five trips for two to any of the following **chocolate capitals**: Switzerland, Holland, West Germany, France, and Ivory Coast.

- **Chocolate courses** are often available through local adult education and/or confectionery kitchens. Richardson Researchers, Inc. of Hayward, California, offers three courses for five days each: Confectionery Technology, Chocolate Technology, and A Short Course in Continental Chocolates.

- **Chocolate of Course** is a service out of Seattle that will deliver goodies to you and/or your friends each month.

- The National Society of Chocolate Lovers sponsors a **Chocolate Cruise to Alaska** out of Vancouver, British Columbia. You are greeted with a basket of chocolates in your stateroom, participate in a truffle taste-in, have lessons in creating, cooking, and consuming chocolate, play chocolate games, and eat chocolate while you cruise for the whole week.

- "There's plenty of talk about the ever-growing **chocolate cult,** but most people have never even tasted real chocolate," according to Thomas Krön, founder of Krön Chocolatier. The secret of true chocolate, he says, is in the cocoa butter.

- As part of a promotion to attract advertisers, *Chocolatier* magazine hired Gerald Schwartz of Gerel Chocolatier to make 20,000 hand-dipped Chinatown **chocolate fortune cookies** with quotes and statistics about the growing chocolate industry.

- Galerie Au Chocolate in Cincinnati offers a **chocolate-of-the-month** gift plan.

- **"Chocolate Spoken Here"** is imprinted on an apron made by Silver Designs of Seattle, Washington, in English, French, German, Hebrew, Italian, Japanese, Norwegian, Polish, and Spanish.

- Hershey's and Reese's ran a **"Christmas Keepsake Offer"** of a Hershey's Elf for a required number of proofs of purchase.

- Cadbury offered **"Clovis the Cow"** hand puppet–a good way for them to promote their use of dairy milk in their chocolate. Another Cadbury promo has been the Country Milk Tin.

- Chocolate Chocolate of Washington, D.C., a division of Park, Ltd., offers a **corporate discount program** of Swiss chocolates at a savings of 35% to 50% off retail.

- *Better Homes and Gardens* magazine recently ran a **"December Fancy Chocolate Desserts"** contest where winners would receive money, a framed certificate of endorsement, and six printed copies of their recipe.

- The Sahara Hotel in Las Vegas sponsored a highly successful **"Discovery Chocolate Weekend"** last spring.

- Falcon Travel of San Diego offers a **European Chocolate Adventure**; its target market: chocophiles, chocoholics, chococonnoisseurs, chocolovers, or chocomaniacs.

- Your **"face in chocolate,"** the theme of Chocolate Photos of New York, has innumerable applications, according to its president, Victor Syrmis. They also do chocolate logos.

- About 65% of American candies have been around for more than **50 years**; it's difficult to introduce new brands into the top 20.

- Bailey's of Boston has kept **file cards** of its customers' preferred chocolate assortments throughout its century-old existence.

- At one point Americans could order **Godiva chocolates delivered** by a woman resembling the company's namesake: long, light hair cascading over a flesh-colored body suit, riding a white horse, and escorted by minstrels. The delivery charge was close to $3,000.

- For 12 wrappers from their various candy bars, Hershey's **"Great American Free-For-All"** offered 5,000 Sony Walkmans, 10,000 Hershey's backpacks, and a free Hershey's painter's cap for all entrants.

- **Hammerheads Restaurant** in Monterey, California, near Fisherman's Wharf and Cannery Row, offers all-chocolate desserts that can be eaten with a meal or a la carte.

- When chocolate maker John **Hannon** of Ireland came to the United States and decided to join forces with Dr. James Baker of Dorchester, Massachusetts, they set up what is today the oldest chocolate company in the country. Their 1777 advertisement read:

> Hannon's Best CHOCOLATE
> Marked upon each cake J.H.N.
> Warranted pure, and ground, exceeding fine.
> Where may be had any Quantity, from 50 wt. to
> a ton, for Cash or Cocoa, at his Mills in Milton.
> N.B. If the Chocolate does not prove good, the
> Money will be returned.

- **Hershey's Chocolate World** in Hershey, Pennsylvania, accommodates up to 16,000 people a day. Automated cars take tourists through scenes of the complete chocolate process, beginning with harvesting the cocoa beans and ending with chocolate being made into a Hershey Bar.

- **Hofstra University** of Hempstead, New York, ran a Chocolate Conference in December of 1988. Some of the academic papers presented, among others, were:

  1. Leon Schiffman (CCNY, Marketing Dept.)–"Kids and Chocolate"
  2. Maurice J. Elias (Rutgers, Psych.)–"Choctelligence: The Missing Ingredient in Educational Reform and Children's Mental Health"
  3. William A. McIntosh et al. (Texas A&M, Sociology)–"Chocolate and Loneliness Among the Elderly"
  4. Andrew T. Weil (UAriz, Medicine)–"Women and Chocolate"
  5. Charles L. Levinthal (Hofstra, Psych.)–"Chocolate on the Brain: Research from the Field of Neuroscience"
  6. Larry M. and Elena Rose Starr (Villanova, Psych.)–"Locus of Control and Chocolate Perceptions"
  7. Catherine S. Elliott (William & Mary, Eco.)–"Rational Chocolate Addiction or How Chocolate Cures Irrationality"
  8. Alice Ross (SUNY/Stony Brook, History)–"A History of Chocolate"
  9. Alex Szogyi (Hunter, Romance Lang.)–"Chocolatissimo!"
  10. Marion Nestle (NYU, Home Ec.)–"The Role of Chocolate in the American Diet: Nutritional Perspectives"
  11. David M. Nathan (Harvard, Diabetic Research Center)–"Exploding Nutritional Myths: The Bittersweet Truth of Chocolate and Diabetes"
  12. Charles S. Telly (SUNY/Fredonia, Business)–"Chocolate–Its Quality and Flavor"

- Nestle sponsors an **International Chocolate Tour** that allows a specified number of gifts from different countries each year for "friends, relatives, and business associates."

- In its November 1984 issue *National Geographic* featured "Chocolate: Food of the Gods." Author Gordon Young cites a manufacturer of the multibillion-dollar industry as declaring, "I'm dealing in pure **joy**."

- **"Luxury chocolates,"** according to Nestle's "Boxed Chocolate Market" study, have become an increasingly important market sector. Purchasers are profiled as people who prefer "impressive" brands, are slightly younger and more affluent, and are more likely to buy chocolates for more personal occasions than for general holidays.

- Mauna Kea Beach Hotel in Kamuela, Hawaii, offers a one-pound box of chocolate-covered **macadamia nuts**.

- Nestle offers a **"Morsels Doll"** (P. Nutty, Scotchy, Semi-Sweetie, L'il Bits, and Milky) free with proofs of purchase of Nestle Morsels.

- **Morty Morsel**, a giant chocolate chip, was recently created for the 50th anniversary of the Nestle Toll House Morsel. Standing five feet tall, five-and-a-half-feet wide, and weighing 3,000 pounds, Morty had to be hoisted by crane onto a second-floor Manhattan loft for the celebration.

- Snickers and M&Ms were designated the official snack foods of the 1984 **Olympics**.

- "A **passion for chocolate** is spreading in the United States as quickly as a dark bittersweet truffle melts on the tongue. Local supermarket racks that once held only Hershey, Whitman's Samplers, and an occasional Nestles Crunch now are crammed with Toblerone bars, Lindt's exotic fruit-filled confections, Cadbury's dipped graham crackers, and bittersweet Droste apples."

  –Mary Alice Kellogg, *Signature* (February 1983)

- Driessen Chocolates of the Netherlands are laden with **patriotic pride**: they are packaged with blue Delft tiles depicting Dutch windmill scenes, and are embossed with the national insignia.

- Betty Furness, commenting on NBC's *Today Show* (January 10, 1985) about how gooey chocolate desserts on the covers of magazines greatly influence sales, reflected, "Never underestimate the **power of chocolate**."

- Melvin Schecter, President of the Chocolate Letter, is trying to convince businesses to send out **chocolate promotional messages** in conjunction with their logo: "A sales message printed on paper can be easily thrown away without being read, but chocolate, that's something people take seriously."

  –quoted in (Springfield, Massachusetts) *Daily News*
  October 10, 1984

- Nestle has produced a number of **recipe books** that it gives free for Nestle Morsels purchases. Some examples are "Candy Craft," which uses Nestle's milk chocolate morsels, and "Sweet Celebrations!" that includes its Little Bits and semisweet morsels.

- **Ronsvalle's Candies** of Syracuse, New York, offers lectures to local churches, clubs, and organizations. Gladys Ronsvalle says they also offer free samples of their more than 200 kinds of chocolates, which "make you turn into a little girl or boy again!"

- Hershey's/Reese's is running a **"Scholar Dollars"** sweepstakes for $365,000 in United States Savings Bonds. No purchase is necessary; details are on their products.

- Swiss Miss recently sponsored a "Chocolate Lovers" **sweepstakes** with five grand prizes of TWA Getaway Vacations to the chocolate capitals of Europe.

- **SwissAir** ran a very effective advertisement depicting 100 labeled chocolates that it serves its First Class passengers. The enticement is titled: "A very exalted brand of Swiss chocolates, generally found at an altitude of 12,000 meters." The airline offers Chocolate Lovers Tours of Switzerland (800/777-9480).

- The **Swiss National Tourist Offices** in New York, San Francisco, and Toronto have lists of chocolate factories that can be contacted regarding tours. The Consulate General of Switzerland keeps track of Swiss chocolate importers.

- Here is the way Journeyworld of New York describes its Chocolate Lovers Tour of **Switzerland**: "Travel at a leisurely pace through spectacular countryside; dine on superb cuisine; stay at elegant hotels; sightsee medieval towns and picturebook villages and make exclusive visits to the chocolate plants of Lindt, Tobler, and Suchard to learn the secrets of great chocolates and sample innumerable varieties to your heart's content."

- A **tavern sign** near Salem, Massachusetts, in the mid-eighteenth century read:

    > Francis Symonds Makes and Sells
    > The best of Chocolate, also Shells.
    > I'll toll you if you have need
    > And feed you well and bid you speed.

- **Chocolate trade** organizations include:

    1 England–Cocoa, Chocolate and Confectionery Alliance, London
    2. France–Chambre Syndicale National des Chocolatiers, Paris
    3. Mexico–Conadeca, Tlaxcala
    4. Switzerland–Chocosuisse, Bern
    5. United States–Chocolate Manufacturers of America, McLean, Virginia

- The oldest grocery **trademark** in the United States is claimed by Baker's Chocolate: "The Beautiful Chocolate Girl," Anna Baltrauf. The story has it that she was working in a Viennese chocolate shop in 1745 when she met Prince Ditrichstein, an Austrian nobleman who fell in love with her and asked her to marry him. When the new bride's portrait was commissioned, it was decided to have her dressed as she was when they met. The painting was seen in the Dresden Gallery by the president of Baker's Chocolate in 1862, and he decided to adopt it as the company's symbol.

- Boston's Copley Plaza Hotel sponsored a Chocolate Binge for one of its **"Uncommon Weekends,"** conducted through the services of Susan G. Berk's Uncommon Boston, Ltd. Participants toured and sampled Godiva at Copley Place, Thornton's English Chocolate Shop, Neuchatel at the Weston Hotel, whiskey truffles at Rudi's, Dutch Cottage Chocolates, Il Dolce Momento, ice cream and hot fudge at Emack & Bolio, and ended up sampling chocolate liqueurs.

- Many traditional chocolate makers are **upgrading** their candy bars. Hershey, for example, has introduced Big Block, the Golden Almond Bar, and Special Dark for $1. This year it brought out "bite-size immortality" in its Golden Almond Solitaires.

- James **Wadsworth** includes this quatrain in his "A Curious History of the Nature and Quality of Chocolate":

    'Twill make Old women Young and Fresh;
    Create New Motions of the Flesh,
    And cause them long for you know what,
    If they but taste of chocolate.

- Guests with the best chocolate recipe for Hyatt Regency's "Chocolate Addict" weekends win their **weight in chocolate**.

- Chocolate Gallery of New York, a subsidiary of Ultra Cosmetics, offers **chocolate workshops**, including supplies.

CHOCOLATE PSYCHOLOGY

- Gloria Levine, owner of Aphrodite Confections of Love in Huntington, California, credits chocolate with curing her **agoraphobia** (fear of being or traveling in open spaces): "There were no candy stores in Balboa Island I could walk to, so I rented a store. Then I couldn't find candy I liked, so I made my own." Within 18 months, her chocolates were winning national awards.

    –quoted in *Los Angeles Times* (May 15, 1983)

- According to a Lindt press information kit, "Like love, chocolate has never been out of style. Today, Americans consume half the chocolate produced in the world. The chocolate bar is an edible **American flag**, a security blanket for the distraught, a barometer of a healthy nation, a consuming passion."

- Madame de Sevigne (1626-1696), in one of the many famous letters to her daughter, Francoise Marguerite, Contesse de Grignan, wrote: "I took chocolate night before last to digest my dinner, in order to have a good supper. I took some yesterday for nourishment, so as to be able to fast until night. What I consider **amusing** about chocolate is that it acts according to the wishes of the one who takes it."

- In answer to the question, "Is chocolate an **aphrodisiac?**," English writer Helge Rubinstein's *Ultimate Chocolate Cake and 100 Other Chocolate Confections* (Congdon and Weed, 1983) says chocolate is said to generate, "in those who relish it, a complacent and yielding disposition."

- Dr. Susan Schiffman, Professor of Psychology at Duke University, lists three factors in chocolate that make it **appealing**:

  1. Pyrazines, which work on the brain and emotions together in "the pleasure center." Chocolate's good smell is a stimulant in its appeal.
  2. High fat content, which makes you feel full and satisfied.
  3. Carbohydrates, which work on the serotonin in the brain to give you a sense of well-being.

Schiffman concludes: "So, you're stimulating the pleasure centers of your brain, you're making your stomach feel as though it's really full, and you're raising the levels of serotin in your brain. In addition, the sweet taste also sends stimulation up to the taste center which will ultimately end up in the pleasure center of the brain as well."

–Unpublished article by Carol Frakes,
freelance writer in Boston

- Milton Zelman, publisher of *Chocolate News*, remarks, "The more interesting the person and the more dynamic the personality, the more one seems attached to **bittersweet chocolate**."

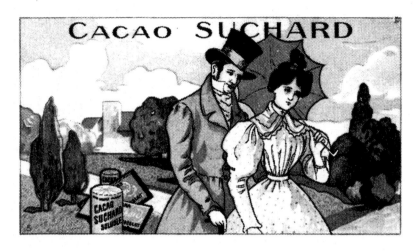

- "Throughout history, giving someone something to eat has been a strategy of control. **Chocolate is magic.** Now when you give chocolate to someone, you want that someone in your power."

  –Jennie Keith, anthropologist (quoted in *Time*, July 12, 1982)

- Jeff Fields of Les Anges in Los Angeles shares his preferences in *Chocolatier*'s Premier Issue: "I like chocolate best late at night. Chocolate is so intense and powerful in taste. At the end of the day I'm really ready for it. It's especially good with champagne. Actually, I find **chocolate and champagne** the adult equivalent of cookies and milk."

- At a Chocolate Festival held at the Fontaineblue Hilton in Miami, a **Chocolate Counselor** was on hand, asking participants: "Do you feel that at times your intense desire for chocolate controls you?"

- **Craig Claiborne,** food editor of the *New York Times*, claims that chocolate is the only flavor the mere mention of which can make Americans salivate.

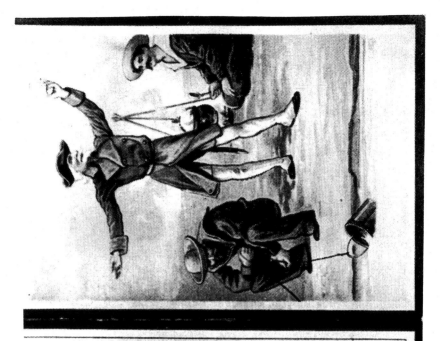

- "What makes you feel good, tastes good, gives you a lift, releases tension and is a counter agent to misery? Why, chocolate–or so it is **claimed**."

  –Bo Niles, *Country Living* (February 1983)

- It has been posited that the first person to eat an oyster was second in **curiosity** only to the first one to bite into a cocoa bean.

- "Chocolate is **downfall**, happiness, pleasure, love, ecstasy, fantasy"–according to Madame Chocolate's *Book of Divine Indulgences.*

- "If I were an anthropologist, I'd say it was cannibalism" says psychiatrist Victor Syrmis of his "Chocolate Photos" business, "but the idea of **eating the chocolate image** of a loved one is very Freudian. Our first contact with the world is oral. Chocolate is made with mother's milk, it's warm, sweet and melts at body temperature. The impulse is to incorporate that person into your system."

  –*US* (September 12, 1983)

- *Snack Food* magazine was told by Professor Joan Gussow of Columbia University that, "This country is going through an enormous **emotional trauma**, and people don't know what to believe. Therefore, we're very susceptible to things we can trust– like a little chocolate chip cookie we can actually see coming out of the oven."

- Susan Heller Anderson records (*New York Times*, December 17, 1980) that, "When chocolate was introduced in Spain in the sixteenth century, it **excited passions and curiosities**."

- "Chocolate lovers do not need any **excuse** for eating chocolate. People eat chocolate for a lot of different reasons. Most simply enjoy the rich, intense, delicious flavor of chocolate. They love the impact it makes on all their senses. Others use chocolate as a reward, while some consider it to be an expression of love or affection"–says Patricia Cobe (*Chocolatier*'s Premier Issue).

- Chocolate brings to mind, according to Madame Chocolate, marvelous **gratification**:

  Children . . . relish it
  Lovers . . . share it
  Chocoholics . . . stash it
  Stockbrokers . . . dabble in it
  Wealthy people . . . lavish in it
  Pregnant women . . . crave it
  Designers . . . market it
  Women . . . need it
  Sensualists . . . indulge in it
  Pagans . . . worship it
  Hedonists . . . enjoy it
  Everyone . . . eats it

- "Chocolate is by nature rich, sensuous, luxurious–all things sinful. And where there is sin, is sure to follow **guilt**," says Julie Davis of the *Los Angeles Times* (October 30, 1985). "The answer to enjoying chocolate without guilt is to recognize that it is a treat, a passion, a satiable desire, and to moderate it so that you minimize any negatives and maximize your pleasure."

- "Few people care who St. Valentine was or what he did to be a saint, but everybody cares what's inside that **heart-shaped box**.
  So if you want her heart aflutter, her pulse pounding and her mouth watering, give her chocolate. (If your Valentine is a he instead of a she, the same trick works just as well.)
  That's because chocolate is not really a flavor, it's a passion–one that some argue is specifically designed to get the hormones dancing, raise the goosebumps and set the spine tingling."

  –Gail Perrin of the *Boston Globe* (February 6, 1985)

- Bob Mannix, Director of Sales for Lindt-Sprungli, says, "We pop the product in their mouths and they're **hooked**."

- A group of researchers from the California School of Professional Psychology in Los Angeles recently compared confessed chocolate addicts and a random sample of other people and concluded: "Those who self-medicated with sweets or chocolates were more likely to have personality traits associated with **hysteroid dysphoria** (an unusual version of depression) and are more likely to be female. Self-medication occurred most commonly in response to depression and tension." Hysteroid dysphoria traits typically include a tendency for unstable moods, an easy tendency toward falling in love, and a feeling of devastation from romantic rejection.

- *Advertising Age* (September 27, 1984) remarks: "Chocolate isn't candy anymore. It's **lifestyle**. It's not just for kids, tugging at their parent's sleeve in the local drug store. It's for a new breed of snobs and neo-epicureans.

  As they say in the chocolate boutiques, chocolate has cachet."

- Defining the **"luxury chocolate buyer"** as one who reports paying at least $10 for his/her purchase of chocolate, J. K. Fuchs and Associates profiles them as:

  - 28-38 in age
  - household income of $25,000+
  - educated–at least some college
  - likely to be childless
  - lives in a two-person household
  - market composition: 61% female, 39% male

- Gastronomic historian and philosopher Brillat-Savarin allows that, "If any man has drunk a little too much deeply from the cup of physical pleasure; if he has spent too much time at his desk that should have been spent asleep; if his spirits have temporarily become dulled; if he finds the air too damp, the minutes too slow, and the atmosphere too heavy to withstand; if he is obsessed by a fixed idea which bans him from any freedom of thought; if he is any of these poor creatures, we say, let him be given a good pint of amber-flavored chocolate . . . and **marvels** will be performed."

- "Ninety percent of the chocolate sold in America is diluted with **milk**, a taste strongly evocative of childhood. It is no coincidence that the nation which created the Playboy bunny also is the home of the chocolate bunny; Americans can enjoy sin only by pretending they are back at an age when they were supposed to know better. The See's chain of 204 stores, widely reported as one of the best of the mass bonbon makers, has thrived by reassuring its customers that 'Mother says it's OK'; the shops are hung with pictures of innocent babies and of Mary See, the founder's mother."

–*Newsweek* (April 4, 1983)

- *Newsweek* continues: "The **need for chocolate** has driven people into the street at 3 in the morning, in search of an all-night newsstand which might stock a Snickers bar. It has led them to do shameful things, like the woman who appeared at Thronberg's shop with a perfectly wrapped gift box she had bought a week earlier for her father's birthday, explaining that she had figured out how to get into the box from the bottom and emptied it herself. 'It's embarrassing,' says Cynthia L., a mental-health worker who eats as much as a pound of chocolate a day. 'Everybody's into health food; everybody's into jogging, and I'm into chocolate.' "

- "If chocolate is your favorite flavor, you are entirely **normal**. It is remarkable how general the taste for chocolate is–how persistent the desire for it. Just ask the boy at the soda fountain how the orders run. He will probably tell you what we have found to be an average for the country. Six of every ten sodas are chocolate flavored. And if the men's preference only were considered, the count would go still higher."

–"Famous Recipes for Baker's Chocolate
and Breakfast Cocoa," 1928

- Chocolate contains **phenylethylamine**, a natural chemical substance that is identical to the one present in the brain that is said to be released when people fall in love or are infatuated. Its presence in chocolate has led some people to believe that consuming chocolate can replicate the physical effects of falling in love. If you want to research this topic further, here are some early studies:

1. Dr. Donald F. Klein and Michael R. Liebowitz, "Hysteriod Dysphoria," Psychiatric Clinics of North America, Vol 11, #3 (December 1979)
2. Dr. John Money, "Love and Love-Sickness: The Science of Sex, Gender Difference and Pair-Bonding," Johns Hopkins University Press, 1980

Of course it is controversial as to whether the phenylethylamine in chocolate actually has any effect, or whether the spurned or heartbroken lover is using chocolate as a psychological form of self-medication. Still, researchers at the New York State Institute have observed lovesick patients craving chocolate emotionally who were soothed after eating it. So much for euphoria!

- Hanspeter Meyer, Vice President for International Marketing at Lindt & Sprungli, labels chocolate as, "a **pick-me-up**. It consoles. Chocolate is a very intimate product."

- Manhattan nutritionist and radio show personality Jackie Storm describes women's intense periodic cravings for chocolate as being part of a **premenstrual** symptom. "Granted, chocolate is high in fat and calories, and women are hungrier than usual a day or two premenstrually, but there seems to be more to this craving than just a need for calories." (*Women's Sports & Fitness*, 12/88)

- Excerpting from its 1945 publication "Food of the Gods–the Story of Cacao," Ambrosia Chocolate Company declares how "chocolate is the **prize** a child receives for being good."

- Sandra Boynton offers different chocolate **profiles** and their chocolate choices in *Chocolate, The Consuming Passion* (Workman, 1982):
  1. The Pastoral Chocolatist–milk chocolate
  2. The Genteel Theobromian–sweet and semisweet chocolate
  3. The Refined Palette–bittersweet
  4. The Sensuous Chocophile–any chocolate
  5. The Vanilla Personality–white chocolate

- It has been repeatedly observed that although chocolate is not a physically addictive substance, some people have been known to develop a **psychological dependence** on it.

- According to a study on stress performed by Dr. Louise Little, Associate Professor of Food Science and Human Nutrition at the University of Delaware, "Chocolate is the food that women reach for most often to **relieve stress**. The women who used chocolate as the food of choice when responding to stress were very emotional about chocolate. They were fiercely loyal to certain kinds of chocolate, and spoke of their love for chocolate in emotional terms."

- Marjorie Schuman, Associate Professor of Psychology at the California School of Professional Psychology, describes how some individuals **respond** to depression, tension, and anger by taking care of their needs with sweets: "If a person uses chocolate as a drug, the user may be a kind of addict." (*Mademoiselle*, 2/88).

- "Chocolate is one of the most effective **restoratives**," says Brillat-Savarin in *The Physiology of Taste* (1825). "All those who have to work when they might be sleeping, men of wit who feel temporarily deprived of their intellectual powers, those who find the weather oppressive, time dragging, the atmosphere depressing; those who are tormented by some preoccupation which deprives them of the liberty of thought, let all such men imbibe a half-litre of 'chocolate ambre,' using 60 to 72 grains of amber per half-kilo, and they will be amazed."

- According to William L. Jorgensen, President of Fanny Farmer Shops, Inc., "While we as a nation are paying attention to our health and diet, we still believe in **rewarding** ourselves with treats from time to time."

  –quoted in *Arizona Republic* (November 4, 1984)

- Chocolate is universally acknowledged as the **sexiest** of all flavors.

- Diane Freistat of Double Truffle in Beverly Hills thinks that "Chocolate does all sorts of good things. There's **something about it** that makes you feel good. It has a nice stimulating effect . . . "

- Joan Lipkis, a chocolatier who teaches chocolate classes at her King's Chocolate House in Queens, says, "My classes laugh when I say this, but I do believe that **chocolate talks to you**. You just have to know what it is saying."

- Husband-wife team of Dr. Roy Fitzgerald, a psychiatrist with the Thomas Jefferson University Medical School in Philadelphia, and Dr. Jennie Keith, Associate Professor of Anthropology at Swarthmore College, have conducted **chocolate therapy sessions** for encounter groups whose members reveal–in complete anonymity–their deepest feelings about chocolate.

- In 1624, Joan Franc Rauch published a treatise in Vienna condemning chocolate as a **violent inflamer of the passions**, asking that monks be forbidden to drink it.

- Norman Kolpas, author of *The Chocolate Lovers' Companion*, suggests that of course chocolate can be part of your diet: "That one-ounce bar contains only about 510 calories, more soothing to the cravings of a weight watcher than a whole ton of celery sticks. If you count your calories carefully, why not include among your daily rations that single, small bar of chocolate? Nibble it slowly, savoring it morsel by morsel, and you will not only increase your enjoyment of it but at the same time, start to build some of the **will power** so crucial in weight control."

- "Some deep thinkers see a lesson in all this," muses *Consumer Reports* in its February 1985 article rating chocolate chip cookies. "They trace the popularity of gustatory splurges to an era of high prices and diminishing expectations. The rich dessert, then, is the **Yuppie's consolation** in a world of contracting opportunities."

Chapter V

Chocoquiz

CHOCOQUESTIONS

1. When was the first book on chocolate published?

2. How many copies did Sandra Boynton's *Chocolate, The Consuming Passion* sell?

3. What name did Richard Cadbury go by when he wrote a book about cocoa in 1892?

4. "Schwarzwaldertorte" is what kind of cake?

5. Rosie's of Boston's award-winning brownie is called:

6. When French Silk Chocolate Pie was first introduced in a bake-contest in 1951, it won $_____ for 1st prize?

7. "ICES" stands for:

8. Sacher torte was invented when, where, and by whom?

9. "Baby Ruth" candy bars were named for:

10. Perugina's "Baci" is the Italian word for:

11. What company accounts for most of the boxed chocolate candy in the United States?

12. Who is credited with perfecting solid milk chocolate for eating?

13. Chocolate chips were first introduced in what year?

14. How many chocolate chips does Nestle produce daily?

15. There are _____ chocolate chips in a 12-oz bag.

16. What colleges are associated with fudge?

17. How many Goo Goo Clusters does Standard Candy produce each day?

18. Hershey's Kisses were first made in what year?

19. _____ Hershey's Kisses are produced each day.

20. How much foil wrap is used on each Hershey's Kiss?

21. Each Hershey's Kiss contains how many calories?

22. "M&M" stands for:

23. Of 100 M&Ms, what color predominates?

24. M&M/Mars is a $ _____ business, _____% of the chocolate bar market.

25. Which two companies dominate the 10 best-selling candy bars?

26. Which company makes the chocolate "orange"?

27. _____ are the best-selling candy at theatre candy counters.

28. The #1 best-selling candy bar in the United States is:

29. Toblerone was invented when, where, and by whom?

30. Tootsie Rolls were invented in what year?

31. The first Whitman Sampler made its appearance when?

32. Chocolate chip cookie sales are an annual business of $_____.

33. Ruth Whitman invented chocolate chip cookies when and where?

34. Eskimo Pie was patented when and by whom?

34. Which company is the largest purveyor of premium ice cream in the country?

35. _____ is credited with being the Father of Chocolate Ice Cream.

36. When and where were chocolate houses first fashionable?

37. When did the British Parliament pass a law forbidding the sale of drinking chocolate without a license?

38. In the sixteenth century, 100 cocoa beans would buy _____.

39. Sandra Boynton's breakthrough greeting card said:

40. The chocolate-flavor business in the United States is a $_____ industry.

41. According to the Chocolate Manufacturers Association, chocolate and confectionery industries provide about _____ jobs.

42. When was the first sale of chocolate in the retail market?

43. Whose slogan is this: "It's the great American, great American chocolate bar."

44. Americans spent $_____ on chocolate in 1984.

45. The oldest grocery trademark in the United States is:

46. How many American publications ran feature articles about chocolate from 1979-1984?

47. What American journal carried the first notice of the sale of cocoa and chocolate, and when was it?

48. Bob Greene of the *Chicago Tribune* is credited with starting the national craze for:

49. Which publication calls itself the "World's Favorite Flavor"?

50. _____ is "The magazine for gourmet chocolate lovers."

51. Chocolate first appeared in the cinema when, and in what film?

52. Comic-strip characters Archie, Reggie, Veronica, and Jughead's favorite hang-out was:

53. The first advertisement of cocoa's introduction in England was announced when and where?

54. _____ is considered the classic chocolate-lovers' movie.

55. Which company is the largest industrial supplier of chocolate and confectionery products to the world?

56. _____ began as a cocoa and chocolate enterprise in 1765 "on the bank of the Neponset River at Dorchester, where it falls to tidewater in Boston Harbor."

57. "Factory in a Garden" describes which company's headquarters?

58. Whose motto is "No other shall I have"?

59. Which candy shops are named for the first American to put her recipes into a cookbook?

60. Ghiardelli is owned by:

61. Godiva Chocolatier, which dominates 50% of the luxury chocolate market in the United States, is owned by:

62. Heath Bars were invented in what year?

63. _____ is considered the "Chocolate Giant."

64. Lindt-Sprungli produces _____ tons of chocolate per day.

65. Henri Nestle began his own company in 1866 with what product?

66. Perugina chocolates are named for:

67. Laura Secord is named for:

68. See's candy boxes all contain a cameo of whom?

69. Who built the first mixing machine for chocolate?

70. Tobler-Suchard has $2 billion worth of international sales in _____ countries.

71. The leading manufacturer of dietetic chocolate coatings in the United States is:

72. World's Finest Chocolates has sold _____ chocolate bars.

73. Which cultures are credited with discovering cocoa?

74. The word "chocolate" is said to derive from:

75. Linnaeus called cocoa "theobroma," Greek for:

76. Chocolate was first noted when, where, and by whom?

77. How long was the chocolate secret kept by Spain?

78. When _____ was betrothed to Louis XIV of France in 1615, she gave her fiancé an engagement gift of chocolate.

79. Who invented the cocoa press, and what year was it?

80. In what year did Rodolphe Lindt produce chocolate that melted on the tongue?

81. Who introduced the process for manufacturing filled chocolates?

82. Which country leads the world in cocoa bean importation?

83. Which country leads the world in per capita chocolate consumption?

84. Does chocolate cause acne?

85. If there are 100 to 150 milligrams of caffeine in a cup of coffee, how many are there in one ounce of bittersweet chocolate?

86. Researchers from where found no statistical significance in calcium absorption between those who included cocoa in their diets and those who didn't?

87. One ounce of chocolate contains approximately _____ calories.

88. Chocolate is a complex substance of how many identified compounds?

89. Does chocolate cause tooth decay?

90. _____ wrote a letter to John Adams in 1785 declaring chocolate's superiority over tea or coffee for both health and nourishment.

91. Chocolate can be lethal to dogs because of which ingredient?

92. A 1.5-oz milk chocolate bar contains how many grams of protein?

93. What is the natural substance in chocolate that is reputed to stimulate the same reaction in the body as falling in love?

94. Who wrote a book about his company subtitled "The Face That Launched a Thousand Chips"?

95. What was the key to the Rocky Mountain Candy Factory's success?

96. What kind of chocolate is used in David's Cookies?

97. What chocolatier was a millionaire by age 25?

98. Who invented the conching process?

99. _____ candy bars are named for Forest Mars' mother.

100. Who began a company in Switzerland that today is the world's largest food corporation?

101. Who was the first person to develop chocolate praline?

102. Which chocolate company bought its own cocoa plantation in the West Indies?

103. A sixth generation of the _____ family runs the business.

104. Which company is associated with nautical novelties?

105. "Dutch cocoa" was based on his discoveries.

106. Whitman Chocolates have been a division of theirs since 1963.

107. Who produced the Field Ration D candy bar for FDR?

108. Henry Savage Landor writes of using chocolate in his mountain-climbing ascent of:

109. In 1528 Cortez wrote about "xocoatl" helping a man to:

110. The whitish film that can develop on the surface of chocolate is called:

111. You can use _____ to substitute for 1 oz of unsweetened baking chocolate.

112. Which states allow the addition of alcohol to chocolate?

113. Belgium has an annual chocolate production rate of:

114. _____ was the site of the first cocoa plantations.

115. Which company was the first to produce candy made with 100-proof bourbon whiskey?

116. Where did the first recipe for brownies appear?

117. Who invented the first "chocolate box"?

118. How many chemical compounds have been determined to be in chocolate?

119. When did Christopher Columbus bring cocoa beans to King Ferdinand of Spain?

120. How long is the conching process for premium chocolates?

121. Which company was the first to use modern refrigeration methods in dipping chocolate?

122. _____ claims to be the oldest confectionery store in Switzerland.

123. Which country was the first to use mechanical devices to manufacture chocolate?

124. The world's largest producer of raw cocoa beans for commercial use is:

125. _____ was the world's first combination bar, developed when?

126. Where was the first roadside candy store in the United States?

127. Who first established the position of "Royal Chocolate Maker to the King"?

128. Which company was the first to set up a chocolate mill in the United States?

129. How much milk is used daily by American chocolate manufacturers?

130. How many chocolate morsels are purchased each day in the United States?

131. What is the word for "chocolate" in German?

132. _____ is the world's oldest confectioner still making chocolates by hand.

133. When and where was the site of the first recorded drinking of chocolate in England?

134. What do Parisians traditionally eat in anticipation of April Fool's Day?

135. It takes _____ cocoa beans to produce one pound of cocoa.

136. The highest candy consumption in the United States is said to take place in:

137. When Chocolat Sprungli bought the Lindt factory in 1899, how much did it cost?

138. What was the world's first chocolate bar called?

139. Who set up the first chocolate factory in Switzerland?

140. Which countries follow the United States in chocolate production?

141. _____ produces more chocolate than any other state in the United States.

142. When the University of California at Berkeley offered a course on the botanical aspects of cocoa production, how many signed up?

143. According to the Guinness Book of Records, the world's largest chocolate sculpture was:

144. Bittersweet chocolate is primarily used for:

145. What is carob?

146. Cocoa is the result of removing most of the _____ from chocolate liquor by means of hydraulic pressure.

147. It is thought that cocoa was indigenous to:

148. The cocoa tree belongs to the natural order of "sterculiaceae," a family of how many genera and species?

149. What is "couverture"?

150. Which government agency supplies information on the Definitions and Standards for chocolate and cocoa?

151. How much lower in calories is dietetic chocolate than regular?

152. What separates good chocolate from the average is:

153. Where do the best cocoa beans come from:

154. "Swiss ganache" is:

155. What is "German chocolate"?

156. The legal requirements of milk chocolate are:

157. Who uses "kosher" chocolate?

158. Pralines are named for:

159. What role do pyrazines play in chocolate flavor?

160. What is unsweetened chocolate?

161. Why is "white chocolate" not considered real chocolate?

162. Who included the "Chocoholic's Creed" in her catalogue?

163. Who fantasizes about picking chocolates from a chocolate tree?

164. According to Joan Steuer, what's the difference between a chocoholic and a chocophile?

165. Who declared, "The people who make constant use of chocolate are the ones who enjoy the most steady health."

166. What is chocoholic Katharine Hepburn's favorite form of chocolate?

167. Who is the first recorded chocoholic, and how did s/he earn this title?

168. When Adrianne Marcus, author of *The Chocolate Bible* dies, she doesn't want to be embalmed, but:

169. Who has a collection of 50,000 chocolate-bar wrappers from 93 countries?

170. _____ is said to have owned the most expensive porcelain chocolate serving service ever made.

171. Who wrote a treatise on "Fasting from Chocolate in Lent"?

172. What is "hagelslag"?

173. What is a Mexican "molinillo" used for?

174. Southwesterns like "mole," which is:

175. How do people of the Appalachians like to eat their chocolate?

176. What target audience is most likely to purchase designer chocolates?

177. The week between Christmas and New Year's is known in France as:

178. The Jesuit priest _____ encouraged monks' use of chocolate.

179. The legend about chocolate being an aphrodisiac originates from:

180. Perugina's "Baci" were named in honor of:

181. Who invented the heart-shaped Valentine's Day box?

182. What famous lovers used chocolate as a means of seduction?

183. Nearly _____% of chocolates purchased as gifts are reported to be bought at specialty candy shops.

184. What is the tradition in Japan for Valentine's Day?

185. Who called chocolate "The Indian Nectar"?

186. How is the game "CACAO" played?

187. Who invented chocolate mousse?

188. What is the most popular chocolate liqueur?

189. What was the result of the affair between Peppermint Patty and Mr. Goodbar?

190. Who considered chocolate improper for American tables?

191. What promotion did Suchard use to celebrate its 150th anniversary?

192. Some of the features of Wilbur's Candy Americana Museum include:

193. Who has an extensive collection of chocolate ephemera?

194. Consumer expert Betty Furness has said about chocolate:

195. Name some countries that have chocolate trade organizations:

196. Dr. Susan Schiffman credits chocolate's appeal to:

197. Who has claimed that chocolate is the only flavor the mere mention of which can make Americans salivate?

198. J. K. Fuchs and Associates profile the "luxury chocolate buyer" as:

199. *Chocolate, the Consuming Passion* gives these profiles of chocolate people:

200. Chocolate is universally acknowledged as the _____ of all flavors.

CHOCOANSWERS

1. 1609
2. 600,000 in the United States; 100,000 in the United Kingdom
3. "Historicus"
4. Black Forest Cake
5. "Chocolate Orgasm"
6. $1,000
7. International Cake Exploration Society
8. 1832 in Vienna by Franz Sacher
9. President Grover Cleveland's youngest daughter
10. Kisses
11. Nestle
12. Daniel Peter of Switzerland, in 1875
13. 1939

14. 250 million
15. 675
16. Smith, Mount Holyoke, and Vassar
17. More than 150,000
18. 1907
19. 20 to 25 million
20. 5 square inches
21. 25 calories
22. Mars and Murrie, the company's founders
23. Brown
24. $1.4 billion, 43%
25. M&M/Mars and Hershey
26. Joseph Terry & Sons
27. Raisinettes
28. Snickers
29. 1907 in Switzerland by Theodor Tobler
30. 1896
31. 1912
32. $7 billion
33. 1931 at the Toll House Restaurant
34. 1922 by Christian Nelson
35. Haagen-Daz
36. Montezuma
37. 1690
38. Slave
39. "Things are getting worse–send chocolate."
40. $25 million
41. 300,000
42. 1657
43. Hershey Bar
44. $4 billion
45. Baker's "The Beautiful Chocolate Girl"
46. 68
47. *Boston Gazette* in 1770
48. Canfield's Diet Chocolate Fudge Soda
49. *Chocolate News*
50. *Chocolatier*
51. 1933, *Dinner At Eight*

52. Pop's Choklit Shoppe
53. 1657, *Public Advertiser*
54. *Willie Wonka and the Chocolate Factory*
55. Ambrosia
56. Walter Baker & Co.
57. Cadbury
58. Chocolaterie H. Corne de la Toison d'Or
59. Fanny Farmer
60. Golden Grain Macaroni Company
61. Campbell Soups
62. 1928
63. Hershey Foods
64. 50
65. A unique milk product for infants
66. Italian town of founder
67. Canadian heroine of the War of 1812
68. Mary See
69. Philipp Suchard
70. 100
71. Van Leer
72. 2 billion+
73. Aztec and Mayan
74. Mayan "xocoatl" and Aztec "cacahuatl"
75. Food of the gods
76. 1519 by Hernando Cortez at the court of Emperor Montezuma
77. 100 years
78. Spanish princess Maria Theresa
79. 1828, Van Houten
80. 1879
81. Jules Sechaud, 1913
82. U.S.
83. Switzerland
84. No, according to the AMA and FDA
85. 5 to 10 milligrams
86. University of Illinois
87. 150
88. 300+
89. No, actually has decay-prohibiting property

90. Thomas Jefferson
91. Theobromine
92. 6
93. Phenylethylamine
94. Wally "Famous" Amos
95. Location
96. Lindt
97. Milton Hershey
98. Rodolph Lindt
99. Ethyl M
100. Henri Nestle
101. Jean Jeuhaus
102. World's Finest
103. Sprungli
104. Harbor Sweets
105. Van Houten
106. Pet
107. Hershey
108. Lumpa peaks of the Himalayas
109. Walk all day without food
110. Bloom
111. 3 Tablespoons cocoa plus 1 Tablespoon butter
112. Nevada, Kentucky, Tennessee
113. 135,000 tons
114. Brazil
115. Rebecca Ruth
116. *Fanny Farmer Cookbook,* 1896 edition
117. Richard Cadbury, 1868
118. 1,200
119. July 30, 1502, his 4th trip
120. 72 hours
121. Page and Shaw of Boston
122. Eichenberger
123. France
124. Ghana
125. Goo Goo Clusters, 1912
126. Hebert Candy Mansion, Rt 20, Shrewsbury, MA, 1946
127. King Louis XIV

128. Walter Baker
129. 3,500,000 pounds
130. 240 million
131. Schokolade
132. Neuhaus
133. 1650, Oxford
134. Chocolate fish
135. 2 pounds
136. Salt Lake City, Utah
137. 1.5 million gold francs
138. Surfin
139. Cailler, 1819
140. West Germany, Netherlands, Great Britain
141. Pennsylvania
142. 800+
143. Red Tulip's 10-foot, 4,484-lb chocolate Easter egg
144. Baking
145. Mashed fruit of a Mediterranean pine tree
146. Cocoa butter
147. Forests of the Amazon and Orinoco
148. 41,521
149. A coating chocolate
150. FDA
151. It's not; in fact, it can actually be more caloric
152. Amount of cocoa butter
153. South America
154. Their invention, a combination of the very freshest possible cream and the finest quality chocolate
155. A special blend of chocolate, sugar, cocoa, and butter
156. At least 25% cocoa components, 14% milk, and sugar content not to exceed 55%
157. Jewish dietary laws prescribe them
158. French Duke of Plessis-Praslin, 1671
159. They give it its bitter and nutty taste
160. Pure chocolate liquor with no sugar added
161. Although it has cocoa butter, it has no chocolate liquor
162. Madame Chocolate
163. Maida Heatter

164. Chocophile considers chocolate a gourmet item
165. Brillat-Savarin
166. Brownies–dark, pudding-like brownies
167. Montezuma, for drinking 50 cups of chocolatl a day
168. Dipped–in chocolate
169. Harry Levene of London
170. Madame de Pompadour, mistress to Louis XV
171. Daniel Concuna, 1748 in Venice
172. Dutch chocolate shot
173. Froth up hot chocolate
174. Spicy chocolate dressing for poultry
175. On biscuits
176. East and west coasters
177. "La treve des confiseurs"
178. Acosta
179. Montezuma's drinking it before entering his harem
180. Love affair in 1930s between Giovani Buitoni and an older, married woman; they exchanged love messages via notes wrapped around chocolates
181. Richard Cadbury, 1861
182. Casanova and the Marquis de Sade
183. 50
184. Girls give chocolate to boys, not the other way around
185. Henry Stubbe, 1662
186. Like BINGO, only with cocoa beans
187. Henri de Toulouise-Latrec
188. Creme de cacao
189. Baby Ruth
190. Harriet Beecher Stowe
191. Poster reproduction of an 1898 advertisement
192. Equipment used by early candy makers
193. William Frost Mobley of Wilbraham, MA
194. Never underestimate its power
195. England, France, Mexico, Switzerland, U.S.
196. Pyrazines, high fat content, and carbohydrates
197. Craig Claiborne
198. 28-38 in age; household income $25,000+; educated; likely to be childless; lives in 2-person household; 61% F, 39% M

199. Pastoral Chocolatist (milk choc); Genteel Theobromian (sweet and semisweet choc; Refined Palette (bittersweet); Sensuous Chocophile (chocolates); Vanilla Personality (white choc)
200. Sexiest

Appendix A:
Choco-Marketing-Mania Survey

Company Information

Name:

Address:
  Street/P.O.:
  State and zip code:
  Country:

Telephone number:

Director of Marketing:

History of the company:

Structure (enclose a chart, if possible):

  Board of Directors

  Administration

  Staff

  Departments

Products:

Annual sales:

Distribution channels:

Target populations:

Media resources:

Advertising budget:

P/R activities:

Chocolate Information

1. Do you use chocolate itself as a product?
   (for example: candy, drinks, cakes, cookies)
   ____ No
   ____ Yes
   (If no, Skip to #6)

2. If yes, approximately what percent is chocolate of your business?
   ____%

3. If yes, how much chocolate did you use this last fiscal year?
   ____ (pounds, tons, etc.)

4. What is your annual promotional budget for chocolate products?
   $____

5. Do your future plans include using more chocolate?
   ____ No
   ____ Yes
   ____ Undecided

6. Do you use chocolate as a concept to sell your products?
   (for example: paper products, clothing, humorous notions, etc.)
   ____ No
   ____ Yes
   (If no, this ends the questionnaire.)

7. If yes, what percent of your business is chocolate-oriented?
   ____ %

8. What ways in particular have you used chocolate in your marketing?

9. Do your future plans include using more chocolate as a by-product?
   ____ No
   ____ Yes
   ____ Undecided

10. Further comments:

Thank you very much for your cooperation. Let us know if you would like to have a copy of these results. Please return this survey to:
   Dr. Linda K. Fuller
   499 Main Street
   P.O. Box 264
   Wilbraham, MA 01095
   Tel. 413/596-3539

Appendix B:
Media Citations
Chocolate 1979-1992

Ad Forum
Advertising Age
Adweek's Marketing Week
Americana
American Legion
Americas
Back Stage
Barrons
Bazaar
Better Homes and Gardens
Beverage Industry
Bicycling
Black Enterprise
Boston Magazine
Business Week
Canadian Consumer
Candy Industry
Chain Store Age Executive
Changing Times
Chemical & Engineering News
Chicago
Childhood Education
Chocolatier
Christian Science Monitor
Colorado Business Magazine
Consumer Reports
Cosmopolitan
Crain's Chicago Business

Crain's New York Business
Cuisine
Current Health
Direct Marketing
Discover
Dynamic Years
Ebony
The Economist
FDA Consumer
Financial World
Food Development
Food Product Development
Food Processing
Food Product Development
Food Technology
Forbes
Fortune
Gifts & Decorative Accessories
Good Housekeeping
Gourmet
Harpers Bazaar
Health
History Today
Horticulture
House and Garden
House Beautiful
Independent Restaurants
Instructor
Journal of Commerce and Commercial
Library Journal
Life
Los Angeles
Mademoiselle
Madison Avenue
Management Today
Marketing
Marketing and Media Decisions
Minneapolis-St. Paul

Money
Moneysworth
Mother Earth News
National Geographic
Nation's Business
Nation's Restaurant News
New England Business
New Scientist
New Statesman & Society
Newsweek
New York
New York Times
New York Times Book Review
Packaging
Packaging Digest
People Weekly
Philadelphia
Popular Photographer
Prevention
Progressive Grocer
Publishers Weekly
Reader's Digest
Redbook
Restaurant Business Magazine
Restaurant Hospitality
Restaurants & Institutions
Sales and Marketing Management
San Francisco Business Times
Savvy
School Library Journal
Science News
Seventeen
Smithsonian
Southern Living
Sport
Sunset
Supermarket
Texas Monthly

Time
Town and Country
Trailer Boats
Travel-Holiday
USA Today
U.S. Distribution Journal
U.S. News & World Report
United States Tobacco and Candy Journal
Vogue
Wall Street Journal
Washingtonian
Washington Post
Weight Watchers
Wilson Library Bulletin
Working Woman

Appendix C:
Addresses of Chocolate Companies

Chocolate Companies

Ambrosia Chocolate Company
1133 North Fifth Street
Milwaukee, WI 5320-1094
414/271-2089

Astor Chocolate Corp
48-25 Metropolitan Avenue
Glendale, NY 11385
718/386-7400

Au Chocolat
1962 W 4th Avenue
Vancouver, BC, Canada
604/734-4737

Baker's
General Foods Consumer Center
250 North Street
White Plains, NY 10625

Karl Bissinger French Confections
3983 Gratior
St. Louis, MO 63110
800/325-8881

Blommer Chocolate Company
P.O. Box 45
East Greenville, PA 18041
215/679-4472

Sydney Bogg
18932 Woodward Avenue
Detroit, MI 48203
313/368-2470

E. J. Brach's Sons
Box 802
4656 West Kinzie Street
Chicago, IL 60690-0802
312/626-1200

Peter Paul Cadbury, Inc.
New Haven Road
P.O. Box 310
Naugatuck, CT 06770
203/729-0221

Chambre National Des Chocolatiers
194 Rue de Rivoli
75001 Paris, France

Chandon Chocolates
24 East 66th Street
New York, NY

Chocolate Chocolate
Georgetown Park
3222 M St. NW
Washington, DC 20007
202/338-3356

Chocosuisse/Union des fabricants suisses de chocolat
Munzgraben 6
3000 Bern 7, Postfach 84
Switzerland

COCOA/Chocolate and Confectionery Alliance
11 Green Street
W1Y 3RF London, England

Cocolat
2547-9th Street
Berkeley, CA 94710
415/843-1182

Cocoline Chocolate Company, Inc.
689-697 Myrtle Avenue
Brooklyn, NY 11205
718/522-4500

Conadeca/Comision Nacional del Cacao
Tlaxcala No. 208
Mexico 11

Corne de la Toison d'Or
Rue Auguste Lambiotte 79/81
B-1030 Brussels, Belgium

Cote d'Or
Rue Barastraat 40
B-1070 Bruxelles
Belgium

Dilettante Chocolates
2306 E. Cherry
Seattle, WA 98122
206/328-1530

Double Truffle Chocolates
259 S. Roxbury Drive
Beverly Hills, CA 90212
800/621-7084

Droste Fabrieken BV
Harmenjansweg 129, POB 9
Haarlem, Holland

Elite Israel Chocolate & Sweet Manufacturing Co., Ltd
PO Box 19
Ramat Gan, Israel

Fanny Farmer Candy Shops
4 Preston Court
Bedford, MA 01730

Fanny May
1137 W. Jackson Blvd.
Chicago, IL 60607
312/243-2700

Max Felchlin
Fabrik Fur Die Konditorei
Bahnhofstrasse 63
Ch 6430 Schwyz
Switzerland

Figi's, Inc.
630 South Central Avenue
Marshfield, WI 54449
715/387-1771

Gabrielle's Fine Chocolates
102 West Pleasant Avenue
Maywood, NJ 07607
201/368-1738

Galerie au Chocolat
One Lytle Place
621 Mehring Way
Cincinnati, OH 45202
513/381-3824

Ghiardelli Chocolate Co.
Div. of Golden Grain Macaroni Co.
1111-139th Avenue
San Leandro, CA 94578
415/483-6970

Godiva Chocolatier
701 Fifth Avenue
New York, NY
212/593-2845

Helen Grace Chocolates
3303 Century Boulevard
Lynwood, CA
800/367-4240

Grand Finale
200 Hillcrest Road
Berkeley, CA 94705
415/655-8414

Michel Guerard
Gourmet Resources International
770 Lexington Avenue
New York, NY 10021

Guittard Chocolate Company
10 Guittard Road
Burlingame, CA 94010
415/697-4427

Halba
8304 Wallisellen
Zurich, Switzerland

Harbor Sweets
Box 150
Marblehead, MA 01945
617/745-7648

Hauser Chocolatier
18 Taylor Avenue
Bethel, CT 06801
203/794-1861

L. S. Heath & Sons, Inc.
PO Box 679
Robinson, IL 62454
618/544-3111

Home of the Hebert Candies, Inc.
575 Hartford Pike
Shrewsbury, MA 01545
617/845-8051

Hershey Chocolate Company
19 East Chocolate Avenue
PO Box 819
Hershey, PA 17033
717/534-5337

Holland Food Products
B. P. 150
1500 ED Zaandam
Holland

Hooper's Candies
4632 Telegraph Avenue
P.O. Box 3064
Oakland, CA 94609
415/654-3373

Hooton Chocolate Company
Division of W. R. Grace & Co.
355 North 5th Street
Newark, NJ 07107
201/485-5385

Huwyler
510 Madison Avenue/53rd Street
New York, NY 10022
212/308-1311

Imports Unlimited
PO Box 3065
Peterborough, NH 03458-3065
603/924-9935

Kosher Chocolate Factory
1827 Willow Road
Northfield, IL 60093
312/441-7110

Lenotre Patissierie Traiteur
42 Rue d'Auteil
Paris 75106, France

Chocoladefabriken Lindt & Sprungli AG
8802 Kilchberg
Zurich
Switzerland

Lisa Lerner Chocolates
2984 San Pablo Avenue
Berkeley, CA 94702

Harry London's Candies, Inc.
1281 South Main Street
North Canton, OH 44720
216/494-1118

Luden's, Inc.
200 N 8th Street
Reading, PA 19606
215/376-2981

M&M/Mars
A Division of Mars, Inc.
High Street
Hackettstown, NJ 07840
201/852-1000

Le Chocolatier Manon
872 Madison Avenue
New York, NY 10021
212/288-8088

Madame Chocolate, Inc.
1940-C Lehigh Avenue
Glenview, IL 60025
312/729-3330

Munson's Candy Kitchen
Route 6
Bolton, CT 06040
203/649-4332

Neuchatel Chocolates
1369 Avenue of the Americas
New York, NY

Neuhaus USA
97-45 Queens Boulevard
Suite 503
Rego Park, NY 11374
212/897-6000

The Nestle Company, Inc.
100 Bloomingdale Road
White Plains, NY 10605
914/682-6686

Perugina Chocolates
21 Main Street
Little Ferry, NJ 07643
800/272-0500

Poulain Chocolat Confiserie
B.P. 727 41007 Blois Cedex
B 775 598 816
Paris
France

Rebecca-Ruth Candies
PO Box 64
Frankfort, KY 40602
502/223-7475

Red Tulip Chocolates Pty, Ltd.
201 High Street
Prahran 3181
Victoria
Australia

Regina's Fine Candies
248 So. Cleveland
St. Paul, MN 55105
612/698-8603

Rocky Mountain Chocolate Factory
PO Box 2408
Durango, CO 81302
303/259-0554

Ronsvalle's Candies
205 Cannon Street
Syracuse, NY 13205

San Francisco Chocolate Company
1057 Howard Street
San Francisco, CA 94102

Miss Saylor's Candies
PO Box 16066
Long Beach, CA 90806
213/437-2737

Lee Sims Chocolates
743 Bergen Avenue
Jersey City, NJ 07306
201/433-1308

Laura Secord/Confiserie Smiles Confectionery
1500 Birchmount Road
Scarborough
Ontario MIP 2G5
Canada
416/751-3631

See's Candy Shops
PO Box 5027
Rancho Mirage, CA 92270
619/340-1505

Stork's Chocolates
12-42 150 Street
Whitestone, NY 11357
718/767-9220

Sucrs. de Pedro Cortes, Inc.
GPO Box 3626
San Juan, Puerto Rico 00936
754-7040

Joseph Terry & Sons, Ltd
Bishopthorpe Road
York Yo1 1YE England

Tobler-Sucard USA
1400 E. Wisconsin Street
Delavan, WI 53115
414/728-3403

Sweet Swiss/European Specialties
S. 5013 Dorset Road
Spokane, WA 99204
509/838-1334

E. A. Tosi & Sons Co., Inc.
77 Messina Drive
Braintree, MA 02184
617/848-1040

Toucan Chocolates
31 Wyman Street
PO Box 72
Waban, MA 02168
617/964-8696

Van Houten & Zoon
Beemdelaan PO Box 120
Vaals, Holland

Van Leer Chocolate Corporation
110 Hoboken Avenue
Jersey City, NJ 07302
201/798-8080

Vicki's Fine Chocolates
119 South Sharpe
Cleveland, MO 38732
601/846-1231

Whitman's Chocolates
P.O. Box 6070
Philadelphia, PA 19114
215/464-6000

Wilbur Chocolate Company
48 N. Broad
Lititz, PA 17543
717/626-1131

C & J Willenborg
PO Box 359
565 East Crescent Avenue
Ramsey, NJ 07446
201/825-4300

Willwood Group
Whitestown Industrial Estate
Blessington Road
Tallght
Dublin 24
Ireland

World's Finest Chocolate, Inc.
4801 South Lawndale
Chicago, IL 60632-3062
312/847-4600

Milton York
Milton York Building
Long Beach, WA 98631

Zaanland
c/o Hermetica, Postbux 150
Zaandam, Holland

Chocolate-Related Companies

Boulder Calendar Company
P.O. Box 2066
Boulder, CO 80306
303/444-8878

Chocolate Collection
1717 Van Buren Street
St. Paul, MN 55104
703/790-5011

The Chocolate Letter
130 West 72nd Street
New York, NY 10023
212/666-0428

Chocolate Manufacturers Association of the USA
7900 Westpark Drive, Suite 514
McLean, VA 22102
703/790-5011

Chocolate News
40 West 20th Street, Room 901-A
New York, NY 10011
212/206-0735

Chocolate Photos
200 West 57th Street, Suite 1105
New York, NY 10019
212/977-4340

Chocolatier/Haymarket Group Ltd.
45 West 34th Street, Suite 407
New York, NY 10001
212/239-0855

Coffee, Sugar & Cocoa Exchange, Inc.
Four World Trade Center
New York, NY 10048
212/938-2800

Culinary Center of New York
100 Greenwich Avenue
New York, NY 10011
212/255-4141

Dallas Alice, Inc.
4956 Boiling Brook Parkway
Rockville, MD 20852
301/468-6996

Dreams Come True
5724 Solway Street
Pittsburgh, PA 15217
412/421-8854

Ebullience
125 South Street
Philadelphia, PA 19147
215/625-0244

Hilliard's Chocolate System, Inc.
275 East Center Street
West Bridgewater, MA

Holland Handicrafts
211 El Cajon Avenue
Davis, CA 95616
916/756-3023

Journeyworld Int'l
155 East 55th Street–4E
New York, NY 10022
212/752-8308

Let Them Eat Cake
PO Box 5330
Eugene, OR 97405

Love Chocolate Factory
1010 Maple Street
Hartville, OH 44632

Mohonk Mountain House
Lake Mohonk
New Paltz, NY 12561
914/255-1000

Mauna Kea Beach
Kamuela, HI 96743
808/882-7222

Pink Imports Inc.
145 Reade Street
New York, NY 10012
212/406-9270

Richardson Researches, Inc.
23449 Foley Street
Hayward, CA 94545

Risk Enterprises
P.O. Box 14093
Cleveland, OH 44114
216/226-8383

The Sweet Life, Inc.
14 Princeton Place
Glen Rock, NJ 07452
201/445-2372

Sweet Investments, Inc.
5701 La Goleta Road
Goleta, CA 93117

Sweetvisions Publishing Company
PO Box 49
Newton Highlands, MA 02161

Swiss National Tourist Office
608 Fifth Avenue
New York, NY 10020
212/757-5944

Norm Thompson
PO Box 3999
Portland, OR 97208

UAI Productions
17638 Raymer Street
Northridge, CA 91325
818/886-0257

Uncommon Boston, Ltd.
Sixty-Five Commonwealth Avenue
Boston, MA 02116
617/424-9468

Williams-Sonoma
P.O. Box 7456
San Francisco, CA 94120
415/652-9007

Choco-References

Adler, Jerry et al., "America's Chocolate Binge," *Newsweek* (April 4, 1983): 50+.

Albright, Barbara and Leslie Wiener. *Wild About Brownies*. New York: Barron, 1985.

Alsop, Ronald. "Candy Makers Step Up Fight Over America's Sweet Tooth." *Wall Street Journal* (June 13, 1985).

Ambrosia Chocolate Company. *The Story of Cacao: "Food of the Gods."* Milwaukee, WI: Ambrosia Chocolate Company, 1945.

Ammon, Richard. *The Kids' Book of Chocolate*. New York: Macmillan, 1987.

Amos, Wally. *The Famous Amos Story: The Face That Launched a Thousand Chips*. New York: Doubleday, 1983.

Anderson, Susan Heller. "Making Chocolates in the Artisan's Way," *The New York Times* (December 17, 1980).

Appelbaum, Cara. "Luxury Chocolates Offer Single Serving; Moving Beyond Gifts Could Increase Year-Round Business," *Adweek's Marketing Week*, v.32 (July 1, 1991): 17.

Asquith, Pamela. *Ultimate Chocolate Cake Book*. New York: Holt, Rinehart & Winston, 1984.

Backas, Nancy. "Chocolate mania!" *Restaurants & Institutions*, v.95 (May 1, 1985): 23+

Baggett, Nancy. *The International Chocolate Cookbook*. New York: Stewart, Tabori & Chang, 1991.

Bailin. "What Really Goes on at Chocolate Festivals," *Chocolatier* (May 1988): 32-8.

Baker, Walter and Company. *The Chocolate-Plant (Theobroma Cacao) and Its Products*. Dorchester, MA: Walter Baker and Company, 1891.

Baker, Walter S. *Cocoa and Chocolate: A Short History of Their Production and Use*. 1910.

Baker, Walter S. *Cocoa and Chocolate Exhibits*. Boston, MA: The Barta Press, 1915.

Bangs, Scholer. "California Heavy. Light and Healthy Foods Seem to Reign Supreme, But Regarding Desserts Chocolate Is Still King," *Restaurant Hospitality* (November 1985): 143+

Becket, S. *Industrial Chocolate Manufacture & Use.* New York: Van Nostrand Reinhold, 1987.

Bedell, Thomas. "The Canfield's Report," *P.E.* (February 1986): 18+

Berenbaum, Rose. *Romantic and Classic Cakes.* New York: Irena Chalmers, 1981.

Berger, Lesly. *The Gourmet's Guide to Chocolate.* New York: Quill, 1984.

Better Homes and Gardens (eds.) *Better Homes and Gardens: Chocolate.* 1984.

Black, Sonia. *Chocolate Chocolate Chocolate.* Scholastic, 1989.

Blumenthal, Robin Goldwyn. "Some of Us Have Been Observing Chocolate Week All of Our Lives," *Wall Street Journal* (March 12, 1990): B1.

Boynton, Sandra. *Chocolate: The Consuming Passion.* New York: Workman, 1982.

Brody, Lora. *Growing Up on the Chocolate Diet.* Boston, MA: Little, Brown, 1985.

Broekel, Ray. *The Chocolate Chronicles.* Wallace-Homestead, 1985.

Burum, Linda. *Brownies.* New York: Scribner's, 1984.

Cadbury, Richard (alias "Historicus"). *Cocoa: All About It.* 1892.

Cardenas. *Libro el cual trata del chocolate.* Mexico, 1609.

Charlton, Art. "Chocolate War: Melts in Mouth, Not in Sand," *Union News* (September 27, 1991): 1+

Child, Pauline G. *The 'Exclusively Chocolate' Cookbook.* PGC Publications, 1984.

"Chocolate Bars," *Consumer Reports* (November 1986): 694+

"Chocolate-Chip Cookies," *Consumer Reports* (February 1985): 69+

The Chocolate Manufacturers Association of the U.S.A. *The Story of Chocolate.* McLean, VA: Chocolate Manufacturers Assoc., 1960.

Chocosuisse (Union of Swiss Chocolate Manufacturers). *Chocologie*. Bern, Switzerland: Chocosuisse.

Colmenero. *A Curious Treatise of the Nature of Chocolate*. Madrid, 1631.

Consumer Guide (eds.) *The Perfect Chocolate Dessert*. Publications International, Ltd, 1981.

Cormon, Linda. "America's Enduring Sweet Tooth," *New York Times* (February 21, 1993), F10.

Cormier, Robert. *The Chocolate War*. New York: Dell, 1974.

Crocker, Betty. *Chocolate Cookbook*. New York: Random House, 1985.

Dineen, Jacqueline. *Chocolate*. Carolrhoda, 1991.

Divone, Judene. *Chocolate Moulds: A History & Encyclopedia*. Oakton Hills, 1987.

Douglas, Barbara. *Chocolate Chip Cookie Contest*. Lothrop, 1985.

Dudley, Anderson, and Yutzy. "A Study of Chocolate Consumption Among the General Population: A Research Study," Opinion Research Corporation, 1984.

Echeandra, James and Janette Kitt. "25 by '95: Reaching the Industry Goal" (pounds per capita candy consumption). *Candy Industry* (July 1989): H2+

Egan, Maureen and Penny Ballantyne. *Chocolate Cherry Tortes & Other Lowfat Delights*. Bristol, 1990.

Elkon, Juliette. *The Chocolate Cookbook*. New York: Bobbs-Merrill, 1973.

Ellis, Audrey. *Chocolate Lovers Cookbook*. Exeter, 1985.

Fabricant, Florence, "Cashing in His Chips: David Liederman Puts Big Chunks in His Cookies and Makes a Lot of Dough," *Cuisine* (November 1984): 15+

Felchlin, Max, Jr., "50 Years Pralinosa, 1935-1985." Schwyz, Switzerland: Max Felchlin Schwyz, 1985.

Finsand, Jane. *The Diabetic Chocolate Cookbook*. Publishers Choice, 1985.

Forbes, B. P., "Chocolate and Cocoa," address delivered before the Cleveland Retail Grocer's Association, 1903.

Freedman, Alix M., "Can Chemists Make a Perfect Chocolate? Well, They Try Hard," *Wall Street Journal* (February 5, 1985).

Fries, Joseph H., "Chocolate: A Review of Published Reports of

Allergic and Other Deleterious Effects Real or Presumed," *Annals of Allergy*, v.41, #4 (October 1978).

Frumkin, Paul, "Cookie Chains Cater to Cash-&-Carry Chocoholics." *Nation's Restaurant News* (October 12, 1984): 28.

Fry, J. S. & Sons, "The Manufacture of Chocolate & Cocoa," Bristol: *British Trade Journal* (January 1, 1880).

Fuchs, J. K., "The Chocolate and Gourmet Food Markets: An In-Depth Study," New Rochelle, NY: J. K. Fuchs and Associates, 1983.

Fuller, Linda K., "Choco-Marketing-Mania," paper presented to Popular Culture Association, Louisville, KY (April 1985).

Fuller, Linda K., "The State of the Chocolate Industry," Max Felchlin Seminar, Schwyz, Switzerland, May 1985.

Fuller, Linda K., "Choco-Talk," Holiday Fare's Grand Chocolate Event, The Quadrangle, Springfield, MA, November 1985.

Furland, Alice, "A Passion for Chocolate; the Belgians Lace It With Liqueur, Mix It with Marzipan, and Eat It by the Ton," *New York Times* (July 8, 1990): XX14.

Galvin, Ruth Mehrtens, "Sybaritic to Some, Sinful to Others, But How Sweet It Is!" *Smithsonian*, v.16 (February 1986): 54+

Gonzalez, Elaine. *Chocolate Artistry.* Chicago: Contemporary Books, 1986.

Goodbody, Mary and the editors of *Chocolatier* magazine. *Glorious Chocolate: The Ultimate Cookbook.* New York: Simon & Schuster, 1990.

Greenberg, Hal and Ellen. *Inside Chocolate: The Chocolate Lover's Guide to Boxed Chocolates.* New York: Harry N. Abrams, 1985.

Hadfield, Linda Connell, "Guess which scientific name translated means...'The food of the gods,'" *Current Health*, v.17 (February 2,1991): 22-3.

Hames, Phyllis, "Chocolate by Any Other Color," *Christian Science Monitor* (February 4, 1987): 29+

Hartley, Marilee, "Chocolate: The New After-Dinner 'Mint'; Fine-Dining Restaurants Target the Ultimate Dessert Consumer," *Nation's Restaurant News*, v.18 (October 15, 1984): 1-2.

Head, Brandon. *The Food of the Gods.* London: R. Brimley Johnson, 1903.

Hearn, Michael. *The Chocolate Book: A Sampler for Boys and Girls*. Caedmon, 1983.

Heatter, Maida. *Book of Great Chocolate Recipes*. New York: Knopf, 1980.

Heatter, Maida. *The Ultimate Chocolate Book*. New York: Knopf, 1980.

Hellmich, Nanci, "Goo Goos Grab for USA Sweet Tooth," *USA Today*, (May 7, 1987): 1D+

Henderson, Janice Wald. *White Chocolate*. Chicago: Contemporary Books, 1989.

Henderson, Janice Wald, "A Day in the Life of a Cookie Mogul: Debbi Fields, President and E.E.O. of Mrs. Fields Cookies," *Chocolatier* (October 1991): 48+

Hershey's 1934 Cookbook. Hershey Chocolate Co., 1984.

Hershey's Chocolate Treasury. Western Publications, 1985.

Hershey, Milton Snavely, "There's No Age Limit," *Everybody's Weekly* (October 4, 1942).

Hirsch, Sylvia Balser (alias "Miss Grimble"), *Chocolate Crazy*. New York: Macmillan, 1984.

Hoffman, Mable. *Chocolate Cookery*. New York: Dell, 1981.

Jacobs, Sally, "Competition Is Thick Among Those Selling Expensive Ice Cream," *New England Business* (June 18, 1984): 47+

Johner, Martin and Gary Goldberg. *Mountains of Chocolate*. New York: Irena Chalmers Cookbooks, 1981.

Johnson, W.H. *Cocoa: Its Cultivation and Preparation*. London: John Murray, 1912.

Jolly, Martine. *Le Chocolat*. New York: Pantheon, 1985.

Knapp, Arthur W. *The Cocoa and Chocolate Industry*. Pitman, 1923.

Kolpas, Norman. *The Chocolate Lover's Companion*. New York: Putnam, 1978.

Lambert, Robert. *Fantasy Chocolate Desserts*. San Anselmo, CA: Egozhe Productions, 1988.

Land, Leslie, "Brownies Are the Classic Comfort Food, the Perfect Compensation for a Busy Life," *Self* (March 1990): 138-40.

Lashings, Edwin G. *Chocolate & Chortles*. MTM Publishing, 1975.

Lawrence, Paul A. *In Praise of Chocolate*. PAL, 1981.

Levy, Faye. *Faye Levy's Chocolate Sensations*. Price Stern, 1986.

LOVE: Chocolate Recipes. Beverly, MA: Kristin Elliott, 1977.

Lunzer, Francesca, "Just for the Taste of It," *Forbes*, Volume 134 (October 8, 1984): 211+1.

Maddox, Sam, "U.S. Coming Out of the Chocolate Closet," *Advertising Age* (September 27, 1984): 50+

Magarian, Judith A. and Patricia Horton. *Chocolate Coated Reading*. Enrich, 1980.

Manning, Elise W. (ed.) *Farm Journal's Choice Chocolate Recipes*. Ballantine Books, 1978.

Marcus, Adrianne. *The Chocolate Bible*. New York: G. P. Putnam's Sons, 1979.

Marshall, Janette. *The Alternative Chocolate Book: Carob Recipes*. David & Charles, 1986.

Mayo Clinic Health Letter, "The Sweet and Bitter Truth About Chocolate," *Los Angeles Times* (June 3, 1987): 23.

Melody, Peggy and Linda Rosenbloom. *In the Chips*. Rawson, 1985.

Minifie, Bernard W. *Chocolate, Cocoa, and Confectionery: Science and Technology*, 3rd edition. New York: Van Nostrand Reinhold, 1989.

Mitgutsch, Ali. *From Cacao Bean to Chocolate: Translation of Vom Kakao Zur Schokolade*. Carolrhoda Books, 1981.

Moorman, Ruth and Lalla Williams. *The Seven Chocolate Sins*. Quail Ridge Press, 1979.

Morton, Frederic and Marcia. *Chocolate: An Illustrated History*. New York: Crown Publishers, Inc., 1986.

Myers, Barbara. *Chocolate, Chocolate, Chocolate: The Ultimate Chocolate Dessert Cookbook*. New York: Penguin, 1983.

The Nestle Company, Inc., "The History of Chocolate and Cocoa," White Plains, New York: The Nestle Company.

Nestle Food Corporation, "The Boxed Chocolates Market: A Report on Consumer Behavior," 1983.

Norman, Jill. *Chocolate: The Chocolate Lover's Guide to Complete Indulgence*. Dorling Kindersley Limited, 1990.

Olney, Judith. *Joy of Chocolate*. New York: Barron Books, 1982.

Opinion Research Corporation, "A Study of Chocolate Consumption Among the General Population," a research study conducted for Dudley, Anderson, and Yutzy, May 1984.

Ott, Jonathan. *The Cacahuatl Eater: Ruminations of an Unabashed Chocolate Addict.* Vashan, WA: Natural Products Co., 1985.

Palar, Barbara Hall, "Chocolate: the Deadly Treat for Dogs," *Better Homes and Gardens* (February 1991): 174.

Park, Penny, "Chocolate Checks the Chill that Kills," (chocolate bar, Canadian Cold Buster, designed to combat hypothermia.) *New Scientist* (April 20, 1991): 17.

Parke, Gertrude. *The Big Chocolate Cookbook.* A&W Visual Library, 1968.

Perrin, Gail, "The Sweet Elite: Chocolate's Still King of Hearts," *Boston Globe* (February 6, 1985): 47+

Persinos, John F., "Sugar Baby. Jimmy Spradley's Candy Bar Has Already Charmed the South. Can It Sweet-Talk Its Way into the National Market as Well?" *Inc.* (May 1984): 85+

Prichard, Anita. *Chocolate Candy: 80 Recipes.* New York, Crown, 1985.

Richmond, Tom, "A Tale of Two Companies," *Inc.* (July 1984): 37+

Ricketts, Verne. *Chocolate Fantasies.* Lieba, Inc., 1985.

Rinzler, Carol Ann. *The Book of Chocolate.* New York: St. Martin's Press, 1977.

Roach, Mary, "More Reasons to Love Chocolate," *People Weekly* (February 18, 1991): 57+

Robbins, Carol T. and Herbert Wolff. *The Very Best: ICE CREAM and Where to Find It.* The Very Best Publishers, 1982.

Robinson, Dick, "The Temptation of Chocolate: Need We Resist Any Longer?" *Health,* v.16 (February 1984): 50+

Roth, Geneen. *Feeding the Hungry Heart.* Bobbs, 1982.

Rubinstein, Helge. *The Ultimate Chocolate Cake and 110 Other Chocolate Confections.* Congdon and Weed, 1983.

Running Press Staff (ed.) *Chocolate Lover's Diary.* Running Press, 1989.

Sherman, Elaine. *Madame Chocolate's Book of Divine Indulgences.* Chicago: Contemporary Books, 1983.

Smith, Robert Kimmel. *Chocolate Fever.* New York: Dell, 1972.

Snavely, Joseph Richard. *Meet Mr. Hershey.* Hershey, PA, 1939.

Steingarten, Jeffrey, "Plunging into a World of New Gourmet Foods, Nibbling and Noshing," *Vogue* (October 1990): 306+

Steinhauer, Jennifer, "America's Chocoholics: A Built-In Market for Confectioners," *New York Times* (July 14, 1991): F10.

Stone, Judith, "Life-Styles of the Rich and Creamy," (Chocolate addicts), *Discover*, v.9 (September 1988): 81+

Storm, Jackie, "When Only One Food Will Do," *Women's Sports & Fitness* (December 1988): 22-3.

Tanzer, Marlene, "Choc Talk: Chocolate, Like Speech, Has Regional Variations," *The Morning Union* (September 12, 1984): 28.

Thaler, Mike. *The Chocolate Marshmelephant*. New York: Franklin Watts, 1978.

Tooley, Jo Ann, "Oh, Chocolate" (Consumption of chocolate candy in various countries), *U.S. News & World Report*, v.106 (February 27, 1989): 75.

Tuller, David and Jean Sherman, "Repackaging Chocolates; Chic Boutiques Transform a Snack into a Sophisticated Seduction," *Working Woman*, (January 1987): 45+

Turim, Gayle, "A Bonbon-anza of Beautiful Paper," (William Frost Mobley's collection of chocolate-related antiques). *Americana* (August 1990): 50.

Virtue, Doreen. *Chocoholics Dream Diet*. New York: Bantam, 1990.

Weil, Andrew and Winifred Rosen. *Chocolate to Morphine: Understanding Mind-Active Drugs*. Boston, MA: Houghton Mifflin Co., 1983.

Welch, Adrienne. *Sweet Seduction: Chocolate Truffles*. Harper Colophon, 1984.

Williams, Pam. *Oh Truffles*. Wilmor, 1983.

Wolf, Barbara (ed.) *Beverly Hills Chocolate Recipes*. Beverly Hills, CA: Double Truffle Chocolates, 1985.

Worthington, Jolene et al., "Chocolate in the Kitchen," *Cuisine* (November 1984): 64+

Young, Gordon, "Chocolate: Food of the Gods," *National Geographic*, v.166, #5 (November 1984): 664+

Zisman, Larry and Honey. *The 47 Best Chocolate Chip Cookies in the World*. New York: St. Martin's Press, 1983.

Zisman, Larry and Honey. *Chocolate Fantasies*. New York: Pocket Books, 1988.

Index

Page numbers followed by "n." indicate reference notes.

GAYLORD No. 2005 | PRINTED IN U.S.A.

DATE DUE

GAYLORD No. 2333 | | PRINTED IN U.S.A.